DIET OF HOPE

Your Journey to Health

With every new sunrise, comes the opportunity to

work on your health

Dietmar Gann, MD

Elizabeth Gann, CNC

Copyediting by Two Worlds Branding

Cover design by Caryn Metcalf

Printing by Arizona Lithographers

ISBN 978-0-9848928-1-5

Contents

INTRODUCTION

This book is dedicated to our patients. Our program (Diet of Hope) is based on how we interpret the science of nutrition and what our practical experience has taught us over the last 30 years.

Amazon has listed close to 20,000 books that deal with nutrition and diets. We have evaluated multiple scientific articles, textbooks, expert opinions and popular diet books. Some of the more trustworthy books we have listed in the back of this book. Some of those books cover diametrically opposed opinions. The spectrum of advice goes from low carbohydrate diets to low fat diets, to high protein diets, to whole plant diets, and calorie restricting diets. Then we have the more outrageous claims of a cookie diet, cabbage soup diet, a diet based on a person's blood group and many more. Not only is the public confused, but also the medical profession.

Most physicians believed, or still believe, in the heart healthy diet, a diet popularized with the food pyramid in 1992. We were told we should all eat 6 to11 servings of bread, pasta, cereal and rice daily, starting at age two. In addition, we were told to reduce our cholesterol and fat intake, especially saturated fat and use polyunsaturated vegetable oils instead. Those recommendations originated at the United States Department of Agriculture (USDA), the creator of the food pyramid. The mission of the United States Department of Agriculture is to promote agriculture.

Dr. Willett, professor at Harvard Medical School and chairman of the Department of Nutrition, stated that the USDA food pyramid guidelines are not only wrong, but dangerous. I fully agree with this statement.

Eating saturated fat and cholesterol were thought to be the main culprit causing heart disease. This was a hypothesis that became a universal belief. Eating a low fat and high carbohydrate diet was felt to be heart healthy. The food pyramid was promoted by all medical societies including the Heart Association and Diabetes Association. A tremendous amount of money and effort went into research trying to prove this hypothesis. To date, published epidemiological, biochemical and dietary studies do not support the idea that this type of heart healthy diet prevents heart disease, strokes, high cholesterol or high blood pressure.

Yet, the whole nation adopted the heart healthy diet. Fat consumption decreased, carbohydrate consumption increased. Pasta and cereals became health foods. But this change of our diet had unintended consequences. We are now experiencing an epidemic of obesity and diabetes, plus a multitude of associated medical problems such as metabolic syndrome, hypertension, high cholesterol, sleep apnea, gastric reflux and multiple cancers. These diseases share the same underlying cause: the modern heart-healthy diet. Sixty seven percent of all Americans are either overweight or obese. Close to 100 million Americans have diabetes or are pre-diabetic. The annual cost to society for the treatment of diabetes alone is close to 200 billion dollars.

Death rates for heart disease over the last few years have declined. However, most experts agree that this is related to a very aggressive and successful treatment for coronary heart disease, and not a change in diet. Statistics from the year 2010 show that one million Americans underwent cardiac catheterization, 500,000 patients were treated with coronary angioplasty or stents and 395,000 had bypass surgery. Fifty percent of men over 65 are on statin medications, as are 38% of women. Nearly 50 million adults take blood pressure medications (National Center of Health Statistics). Also, only 24% of adults smoke today compared to 42% in 1965. However we know with the increase of diabetes and obesity there will be an increase of heart disease in the future. The risk of a diabetic patient to develop a heart attack is the same as for the patient who already had a heart attack. It is an official policy that all diabetics should be on statin medications. And so now we have two new expensive medications to treat obesity; we have become more and more dependent on the pharmaceutical industry. Prevention should be the answer for this massive increase of diseases.

I retired from my interventional cardiology practice 3 years ago; together with my wife we are dedicating our knowledge and time to the benefit of our patients. We are convinced, and have data to prove that our program, The Diet of Hope, can help treat and prevent many diseases, especially diabetes and obesity. Our reward: making a difference and changing people's lives.

CHAPTER 1

A CARDIOLOGIST'S JOURNEY

As did almost all of my colleagues, I too believed that a low fat diet would reduce heart disease.

Nutritional classes in medical school were nonexistent. The knowledge a physician receives comes from the same sources available to the public. Primary information is obtained from consensus statements from our government, medical societies and the press. The gospel of the benefits of a low fat diet became ingrained in the national psyche. The popes of nutrition clearly had established a religion: fat and cholesterol were evil. We physicians had no reason to doubt this religion, neither did the public.

As Mark Twain stated, "It ain't what you don't know that gets you in trouble. It's what you know for sure that just ain't so."

There were many diets available, but the consensus was that they didn't work. The pharmaceutical industry was eager to help. The search for a magic pill was intense. Several pills made it on the market (Phen-Fen, Ribonabant), but later one had to be withdrawn because of serious side effects. Now we have two new diet pills. During my career as a cardiologist my philosophy was to prescribe a new drug only after it was tested by the market for at least one year. These two new pills are only modestly effective and very expensive. The Diet of Hope renders much better results

I dispensed the low fat diet advice freely to all my patients. I wasn't very successful. Everybody gained weight; diabetes became an epidemic. Heart disease remained a huge problem. But what else was there?

Dr. Robert C. Atkins started a revolution declaring that the antidote to obesity and diabetes was reducing carbohydrates and increasing protein and fat. Other books were published supporting his thinking, such as Protein Power, the South Beach diet and many more.

This was blasphemy in the eye of the gods of the low fat diet. However millions of people tried these diets and succeeded. Now the patients were teaching the physicians what worked in the real world.

I had my own epiphany when an old patient of mine tried the Atkins diet, lost weight and improved his cholesterol levels. I tried it myself and lost 20 pounds in four months. In spite of eating a high fat and cholesterol diet, my lipid levels improved significantly. I had several discussions with Doctor Atkins; he sent me some of his research results and suggested I do my own research, which I did. This experience made us realize there was life beyond the low fat religion.

Over the next 15 years, my wife and I studied literature on nutrition. My wife became a certified nutritional consultant, and we explored research not just in the US, but also in European countries.

In the nineteenth century, a low carbohydrate diet was generally accepted as a weight loss diet in both Germany and England. The chancellor of Germany Bismarck lost 60 pounds in a year with a diet of lean meat, veal, mutton and vegetables. He avoided sugar, potatoes and limited bread.

Going on a low carbohydrate diet was called "banting" in England. William Banting, a London undertaker, had become very obese; he couldn't tie his shoes anymore. He tried exercise and gained more weight; he reduced calories and felt miserable. He found a physician who introduced him to a diet of meat, fish and game. On this diet program, he lost 50 pounds in a year and felt healthy. In 1863, he published a Letter on Corpulence, addressed to the public.

Doctor Atkins was introduced to a low carbohydrate diet while moonlighting at the Dupont Company when he started his practice. The executives were kept slim and trim on a restricted carbohydrate diet. Doctor Atkins tried this diet himself and lost a significant amount of weight, which convinced him that a low carbohydrate diet was the cure for obesity.

CHAPTER 2

THE DIABETIC CURSE OF MY FAMILY
By Elizabeth Gann

All too early in my youth, I learned about the horrible disease diabetes; a disease that first claims the limbs, eye sight and then life itself. The horror was that "the curse" was in my family genes. The disease was so rampant in my family that no one seemed to question it. It was accepted that each of us was destined to get it at some point.

There was no discrimination. My grandfather got it; my mother was diagnosed with it, and one by one, her brothers and sisters were diagnosed with "the curse". Some got it worse than others and some died too young from the ravages of the disease.

My mother was a very strong, disciplined person. When she was diagnosed with "the curse", she was determined not to let it beat her. The disease had already claimed the lives of several of her siblings, and another had lost his eyesight. She saw the doctor regularly, ate according to the diabetic guidelines and faithfully injected her insulin every morning and evening. I often wondered if that was what was in store for my future. Maybe, if I was lucky "the curse" might skip me. Luck, because it seemed that there was no answer, nor a cure.

I remember on one occasion that my mother's physician found a needle in her foot. Due to the advanced neuropathy in her feet (something that commonly develops in diabetics) she did not feel the needle. Eventually, she developed sores on both her heels after being in the hospital with a broken hip. Somehow, no matter what they did for the sores, they never healed completely. When she was about 75 years of age, we got the dreaded news that her left foot had developed gangrene and her leg needed to be amputated at the knee. I asked myself, why? She had followed all the rules, taken her medication and ate as instructed. Why? What we did not realize was that neither the medication she was taking, nor the insulin, was curing her disease. The medication and the insulin were merely controlling the symptoms of her elevated blood sugar. The disease continued to progress. This was the way "the curse" functioned.

My mother tried to look at the bright side, if there was any, and comforted us by telling us that at least she still had her other leg. That comfort did not last long. , Due to complications, her other leg also had to be amputated. She could walk with her prosthesis, but it was not the same since she had to depend on others for assistance; something that was very difficult for an independent woman. Our father became her main caretaker until she passed away in 2008. After her death I looked around at my siblings and wondered who would be next in line for "the curse".

So what has contributed to the rise of the diabetes curse? Simply put, we believe there is a direct correlation between obesity and diabetes. In the United States, our annual sugar consumption is 170 lbs. per person, a significant increase from 120 lbs. in 1955. We have become a nation of couch potatoes; cooking at home has become a novelty. Even more alarming, as our nephew from Germany pointed out, we have a fast food place in almost every major intersection.

When he said that, I felt insulted. How could he exaggerate that way? Somehow, I felt I needed to refute his misguided notion, so I set out to prove him wrong. Much to my shock, in our neighborhood's major intersection, there are two bagel shops, two hamburger joints, two pizza shops, four restaurants and two ice cream-yogurt shops. What an eye-opening experience. I realized fast food places were so common that I had not even noticed.

So, did I escape the diabetes curse? From our research at the Diet of Hope, I realized the curse can be controlled. While we carry the diabetic genes, they are activated by what we eat.

Our experience with our diabetic patients and my own health is that eating patterns are the determining factor.

"MY HEALTH, MY RESPONSIBILITY"

CHAPTER 3

HEALTH STATISTICS FOR USA FROM THE CENTER FOR DISEASE CONTROL (CDC)

Obesity:

Thirty five percent of US adults are obese with a body mass index over 30%. Non-Hispanic blacks have an obesity rate of 49.5%, Hispanics 39.1% and whites 34.3%. A total of 100 million people are obese out of a population of 315 million.

In 2008, medical costs associated with obesity were estimated at 147 billion dollars because of a higher incidence of diabetes, heart disease, stroke and cancer, especially breast and colon cancer.

Childhood obesity has more than doubled in children and tripled in adolescents in the last 30 years.

The percentage of children age 6 to 11 who were obese increased from 7% in 1980 to 18 % in 2010. The percentage of obese adolescents age 12 to 18 increased from 5% to 18% over the same period. It is very likely that this will be the first generation with a lifespan shorter than their parents.

Diabetes:

Twenty-six million are diabetic with an A1C greater than 6.5%. It is estimated that 7 million people are unaware that they are diabetic. Even worse, 79 million people are prediabetic with an A1C between 5.7% and 6.4%. The complications associated with diabetes start at the prediabetic stage. People age 65 or older have a 26.9% higher incidence of diabetes compared to younger adults. Diabetes is the leading cause for blindness and for kidney failure. Sixty percent of lower leg amputations occur in diabetics, 70% have neurological problems, especially disabling neuropathies; the risk of dementia doubles. Risk for heart disease and strokes quadruple. Estimated diabetes costs in 2012 were 200 billion dollars.

Hypertension:

One in 3 adults is estimated to have high blood pressure (67 million). Only 47% of hypertensive patients have their blood pressure under control. In 2009, 34,800 deaths were related to hypertension. Direct medical costs for hypertension were estimated at 47 billion.

Cholesterol:

Seventy-one million adults are thought to have a high LDL, the bad cholesterol (above 130mg/dl), which represents one third of the adult population. According to medical guidelines, they should be on statin medications. However, less than half of these patients take statins and only half of these patients reach their goal.

Heart Surgery, Bariatric Surgery and Angioplasty:

Annually, close to one million patients undergo either bypass surgery or angioplasty. In 2009, 220,000 patients had bariatric surgery, an increase from 36,000 in 2000.

Breast Cancer:

230,000 new cases in 2009

Colon Cancer:

142,000 new cases in 2007

All these abovementioned diseases we call "Diseases of Civilization." They are related to our present lifestyle and are largely absent in less developed societies. The answers to these diseases are not more medication or surgery. We need a radical change of our thinking and need to openly discuss what went wrong. Solutions are available. We have to be able to stand up to the special interest groups, especially the food and pharmaceutical industries.

CHAPTER 4

DIET OF HOPE

Nearly 10 years ago I first published results of an earlier version of Diet of Hope in the Clinical Journal of Cardiology (Clin Cardiol; 2004 Oct; 27 (10):563-4). Thirty eight of my cardiology patients started on a low carbohydrate diet. They all had serious heart disease and were overweight. When I told them no sugar, bread, cereals, rice, pasta and potatoes for a year, they looked at me and asked what food there was left to eat. What about heart healthy cereals or heart healthy whole wheat? I told them to eat good proteins from meat, fish and fowl. I also advised them to make sure they eat a lot of salads and non-starchy vegetables; use good fats such as olive oil, canola oil, and fatty fish with omega 3 fat and remember portion control. When I told them they could have eggs for breakfast they were incredulous, this was totally against official teaching.

But they trusted me. They had been my patients for years. They followed my advice.

After a year their average weight loss was 31 pounds (range 16 to 107 pounds). Triglyceride levels were lowered by 29.5% and HDL (good cholesterol) increased by 17.6%. These results cannot be achieved by a medication. What is more, none of the patients experienced any heart problems during that year.

It is difficult to spend the time it takes to teach and educate a patient on a proper lifestyle and diet when you have a busy cardiology practice. This is a difficult task for any physician. So, after I retired from my cardiology practice I dedicated all my efforts to create a program teaching proper lifestyle and nutrition to patients and physicians alike. As Albert Einstein once said, happiness is not having all the luxuries in life but being interested in something you can be enthusiastic about. My wife and I are very enthusiastic about our Diet of Hope. Eight years ago, my wife was chosen as the minority businesswoman of the year, a national award. However, the business was not her true calling. She turned over her business to her brother, studied nutrition and became a certified nutrition consultant. The Diet of Hope is about making an impact on those who need us the most.

We studied the nutrition recommendation by our government and realized it was absolutely wrong for the majority of people. Obese and/or diabetic patients do worse on a high carbohydrate diet. Whole wheat is not healthy. For example, animals are fattened with foods high in carbohydrates and humans respond the same way.

Our experience taught us that diabetes can be prevented and sometimes reversed. Common thinking is: once a diabetic always a diabetic. However, people are diabetic or early diabetic because of what they eat. Simply avoiding food that causes diabetes is sufficient. Unfortunately, the food causing diabetes is the exact food recommended by our government. Taking a pill or an injection will not cure diabetes; it's merely a window dressing. Typically, if a patient shows up at a doctors' office and is diagnosed with a disease, the doctor investigates the cause of the disease before he starts any treatment. Diabetics are not evaluated that way; we know what the cause is, but most physicians feel nothing can be done about it. We may as well put the patient on medications. The power of the food and pharmaceutical industry prevents logical thinking.

Fortunately, there is a rapidly growing group of physicians organized in the Obesity Society and the American Bariatric Society. These associations promote a healthy low carbohydrate diet for the treatment of the "Diseases of Civilization," such as obesity, diabetes, heart disease, arthritis, gastric reflux, sleep apnea and many more.

The Diet of Hope is also promoting a similar diet to treat these common diseases. We want the program to be affordable. For this reason, we accept any insurance that accepts us. We help our patients manage their diseases by teaching them proper nutrition, lifestyle changes and behavior modification. Patients on multiple medications need to be medically monitored. Frequently, medications need to be reduced especially in diabetic and hypertensive patients. The primary care physician remains in charge of the overall care of the patient.

We do not use gimmicks, and do not sell any food or medications. On the contrary, we frequently reduce medications used by our patients, especially medications for diabetes, hypertension and cholesterol. One of our diabetic patients was able to save over 4,000 dollars on his yearly medication bill.

Diet of Hope: A Lifestyle Change

- Teaches proper nutrition
- Provides sufficient nutrition
- Teaches portion control
- Prevents hunger and provides satiety
- Makes people accountable
- Helps change behaviors
- Provides daily simple menu ideas
- Avoids simple and refined carbohydrates
- Promotes complex carbohydrates except wheat
- No calorie or carbohydrate counting
- Provides sufficient, but not excessive proteins
- Promotes use of omega 3 fats
- Avoids *trans* fats
- Reduces caloric intake
- Gluten free
- Lactose free
- Aims at reducing prescription drug use
- Ideal for the treatment of obesity
- Ideal for the treatment of diabetes
- Lowers blood pressure
- Promotes health
- Can be followed for life
- No drugs used
- No gimmicks

The Ten Commandments of the Diet of Hope

1. Thou shall not eat the food that enriches the food industry and damages your health.

2. Thou shall eat food in moderation

3. Thou shall eat plenty of non-starchy vegetables

4. Thou shall eat the good fats of the sea

5. Thou shall eat 3 meals a day; each meal will have some protein

6. Thou shall weigh yourself daily

7. Thou shall move your body on a regular basis

8. Thou shall sleep 8 hours a day

9. Thou shall try to involve and teach your family

10. Thou shall listen to your body and not to the sirens of pseudoscience

CHAPTER 5

THE DIET OF HOPE PROVIDES THE BODY WITH ALL THE NUTRIENTS THE BODY NEEDS

Protein:

A complete protein consists of 20 amino acids. Nine of those amino acids the body cannot create; they are considered essential. These amino acids need to be consumed on a regular basis. Most animal proteins are complete meaning they contain all the essential amino acids. Egg protein is complete and easily digested. Many vegetable proteins are incomplete. Vegetarians need to eat a variety of vegetables to receive a complete set of amino acids.

Good Fats:

Omega 3 and omega 6 are essential for the body; they have to come from food. Omega 6 fats can be found in multiple foods, omega 3 fats are mostly found in fatty cold water fish. However, we do not know how much omega 3 fats the body needs. A few grams per day are probably sufficient. People who dislike fish should consider taking fish oil supplements. Oils such as olive oil and canola oil should be part of a healthy diet. Curiously, the new food plate doesn't mention fat at all.

Vitamins:

Deficiency of vitamin C causes Scurvy, deficiency of vitamin D is responsible for Rickets, and Vitamin B1 deficiency causes Beriberi. While we know a lot about our minimum need for vitamins, we don't know what the ideal dose is. Mega doses of vitamins are advertised by the vitamin industry with little scientific support behind their claims. Eggs and meats are full of vitamins. The vitamins meat and eggs do not provide are obtained by the generous consumption of greens and non- starchy vegetables.

Phytonutrients:

Phytonutrients are found in fruits and vegetables. Hundreds of these compounds have been identified and are felt to be important for our health. No standards exist, but eating plenty of vegetables is important.

Carbohydrates:

Our body can function without carbohydrates. There is no known minimal requirement for carbohydrates (Eskimos). The food industry knows how to mix carbohydrates with salt and fat to make the food irresistible and addictive. The business model of the food industry is to hook people on food, which could not be done with natural food. Carbohydrates in the Diet of Hope program come from vegetables and some fruits. They are complex carbohydrates with a low glycemic index.

The Diet of Hope provides all the food the body needs. We generally use no supplements or vitamins, except in patients that have a low vitamin level, such as vitamin D. Also, for patients that cannot eat fish or dislike fish, we suggest they obtain their omega 3 fat from fish oil capsules.

CHAPTER 6

RESULTS OF THE DIET OF HOPE

My wife and I officially started the Diet of Hope over four years ago. Five thousand patients have started our program. Eighty five percent (4,250 patients) were able to finish our phase one program. Phase one is an intensive program. Patients have to be mentally ready to change their lives. The program is not for everyone. Patients are seen on a weekly basis. They are instructed what to eat every day. The food is simple and easy to prepare. For many patients who were accustomed to eating out for every meal, phase one is an adventure that expands their food horizon. During the first few days, patients addicted to carbohydrates may have some withdrawal symptoms.

Weight loss for patients who finish the six weeks ranges from five to seventeen percent of body weight. Weight loss is highly predictable. For this reason, patients who do not lose weight, we instruct them to read the diet instructions again. Weight loss is just a number; however, the health of our patients improves significantly, and sometimes dramatically. For example, patients' personalities may change, they have more energy, diffuse body pains decrease, gastric reflux improves, they sleep better and their brain seems to function better. Many patients return to thank us for giving them their life back. Our Nurse Practitioners call our office "The Happy Place."

What Happens after 6 Weeks?

Being successful in the first 6 weeks provides an enormous psychological boost to most patients. They understand the concept of the plan, they feel better; they suddenly are in control of their weight and their health. They want to continue, but intermittently they still need some support. Initially, we felt 6 weeks was all patients needed, but because of our patients' demands we created phase two and three.

Phase two of the program allows an increased consumption of good fats, fruits and occasionally a splurge meal (food patients crave).The overwhelming majority still need to lose more weight. This program is very individualized. Interestingly, Medicare now allows 22 visits per year to our clinic as long as the patient shows progress. The administrators of Medicare realized that old habits and food addiction cannot be changed long term with a few visits. Intensive behavioral treatment is part of our program.

Results after One Year:

Seventy two percent of patients either maintain their weight loss or lose more weight. Hundreds of patients lost more than 25 pounds. Three dozen patients lost more than 100 pounds, and our star patient Linda lost over 200 pounds.

Twenty six percent of patients gained some weight back, but never regained their previous weight. Some of those patients ask for another 6 weeks of phase one, feeling they needed the accountability and support.

Only two percent of our patients regained all their weight or sometimes more.

Phase Three:

Patients have reached their goal. They will be monitored on an "as needed" basis. Usually they are monitored once a year.

CHAPTER 7

DIET OF HOPE IN THE TREATMENT OF INSULIN DEPENDENT, TYPE 2 DIABETIC PATIENTS

Ninety six insulin dependent, type 2 diabetic patients successfully finished our 6 week program (phase 1).

To avoid hypoglycemic and hypotensive reactions, temporary changes of medications are necessary. Some patients need a substantial reduction in their insulin dose within days of changing their diet.

Changes on Day One:

- We stop regular insulin.
- We stop long acting insulin at night and gradually reduce the remaining dose during the 6 weeks.
- We stop all sulfonylureas (Glipizide, Glimepiride) to avoid hypoglycemic reactions.
- We stop most diuretics. Eliminating refined carbohydrates produces a spontaneous diuresis potentially lowering blood pressure.

- We stop fibrates (Trilipex, Lopid, Fenofibrate). Elevated triglycerides are most of the time related to excessive consumption of refined carbohydrates. Our diet doesn't include refined carbohydrates.

Results:

- Fifty two patients were able to stop insulin completely.
- Forty four patients reduced their insulin dose substantially. Experts say once a patient is on insulin, generally they will always be on insulin. Not true. People are diabetics because of what they eat.
- All patients lost weight. Average weight loss was 25 pounds or 10.3% of their body weight.
- Average triglyceride levels changed from 203 mg/dl to 184 mg/dl or 9%. All eleven patients on triglyceride lowering medications (Fibrates) were taken off the medication.
- Despite of all the reduction of insulin doses, A1C improved substantially. Before the diet was started the average A1C was 8%, at the end of 6 weeks it lowered to 6.8%, a decrease of 15%.

Hippocrates: *Let food be your medicine and medicine be your food*.

Results in Type 2 Diabetics (A1C 6.5 or higher) *not* on Insulin

Nineteen percent of all patients coming to us are non-insulin dependent diabetics. Close to one third of those patients do not take medications, either because they can't afford it, don't want to take medications or are not aware they are diabetic.

- Average weight loss is 9.5% of body weight.

- A1C changed from 7.71% to 6.26%, a decrease of 19%.

Dietary lowering of an A1C is safe. The famous Accord Study of 10,000 diabetic patients showed a higher mortality if diabetic patients were treated aggressively with medications to an A1C below 7%. An A1C number of 7% or above leaves the patient exposed to all the complications of diabetes.

Results of the Diet of Hope in Patients with Prediabetes

Forty one percent of all patients coming to the Diet of Hope are prediabetic with an A1C of 5.7% to 6.4%. Many are not aware of their problem. They came to us primarily of the treatment of obesity. Thirty seven percent are taking Metformin. Diabetes complications start at the prediabetic stage.

Our diagnosis is based on an in-office finger stick test for A1C. An elevated A1C number is a great motivator for our patients to move out of the prediabetic territory.

Seventy five percent of patients with prediabetes are able to normalize their A1C during our 6 week program.

CHAPTER 8

DIET OF HOPE PROGRAM HELPS LOWER BLOOD PRESSURE

One of the common criticisms of the low carbohydrate diet is that patients are really only losing water. This argument obviously doesn't hold up in patients losing 50 or 100 pounds.

There is no question that people on a low carbohydrate diet lose mostly salt and water in their first week, which leads to a lower blood pressure. Rather than asking, why people lose salt and water on a low carbohydrate diet (a good thing), the establishment in favor of the low fat diet, used this finding as a negative.

What is really happening? Insulin not only affects our blood sugar, but also affects the kidney function. High insulin blood levels interfere with our kidneys' normal function and promote salt and water retention. Salt and water retention raises our blood pressure. Lowering the effect of insulin on our kidneys will lower our blood pressure.

Our Results:

Out of our 500 most recent patients, 247 carried the diagnosis of hypertension and were on diuretics and multiple other blood pressure medications.

Systolic Blood Pressure

Average systolic blood pressure:(before the diet)	126.4 mmHg
After 6 weeks:	120.8 mmHg
TOTAL DIFFERENCE:	**4.6%**

Diastolic Blood Pressure

Average diastolic blood pressure: (before the diet)	78.3 mmHg
After 6 weeks:	74.5 mmHg
TOTAL DIFFERENCE:	**4.8%**

The patients' blood pressure before they started our program was obviously well controlled with their medications.

Of those 247 patients, 70 were on diuretics; all 70 patients were either able to stop their diuretics (the majority) or reduce their dose. Seventy-two patients on a variety of other blood pressure medications were able to reduce or stop those medications.

We specifically tried to lower beta blockers, which are known to cause mild weight gain.

Despite of all the reductions in medications during the 6 weeks, patients' blood pressure at the end of the program was still significantly lower compared to the starting blood pressure.

Starting a low carbohydrate diet should be the first step in the treatment of high blood pressure.

CHAPTER 9

CHOLESTROL AND THE DIET OF HOPE

Eating saturated fat and cholesterol has been singled out as the main culprit in elevating blood cholesterol levels and causing heart disease over the last 40 years.

We use statin medications to lower cholesterol. Statins inhibit the function of a liver enzyme called HMG-CoA-reductase. This enzyme stimulates cholesterol production. Insulin stimulates this enzyme and promotes cholesterol production. Lowering insulin levels in our blood lowers cholesterol production.

The effect of the Diet of Hope on cholesterol levels in our last 500 patients:

Cholesterol Type	Starting Level	After 6 Weeks
Cholesterol	184.1	161.4
LDL cholesterol	96.5	88.3
Triglycerides	178.5	142.8

This data show a significant improvement of all lipid levels. All patients on fibrates were taken off the medication at the beginning of the program (11 patients). Twenty one patients were able to lower or discontinue statin medications.

In my opinion, statin medications are over-prescribed. The Diet of Hope program lowers cholesterol levels and is especially effective in lowering triglyceride levels.

The Benefits of the Diet of Hope

1. You will get your health back
2. You are guaranteed to lose weight (fat) if you follow the program
3. Your triglycerides will lower substantially
4. Your good cholesterol will increase (HDL)
5. Your bad cholesterol (LDL) will change to the more benign fluffy form
6. Inflammation in your body will decrease (C-reactive protein)
7. For men testosterone levels will rise
8. Acid reflux will improve
9. Arthritis frequently improves
10. Asthma frequently improves
11. You will feel more energetic and may even want to exercise
12. Your self-image improves, thereby decreasing depression
13. You will not be hungry despite eating half the portions from before
14. If you are a diabetic you will be able to lower some of your expensive medications
15. Despite less diabetic medication your A1C will improve
16. Some diabetics will be able to reverse their disease
17. You take control of your health

Photos of Our Patients

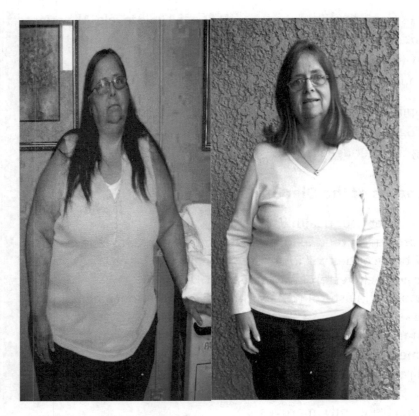

LYNDA OUR STAR PATIENT

Diet of Hope is a lifestyle change of healthy eating. Each day is better than the last. Just believe in yourself, take one day at a time and if you fall off-just make sure and get back on. I had many health problems. My blood pressure, high blood sugar and cholesterol have now normalized. I hope my story inspires many people. Lynda

Over the past 2 years Lynda has lost over 200 pounds.

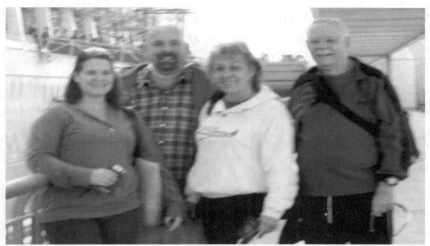

When my wife and I heard about the Diet of Hope and went to the seminar, we thought it was too good to be true. We agreed that we could do anything for six weeks. The rewards were fantastic; my wife is no longer pre-diabetic, I am no longer taking insulin, we lost weight for the first time in our lives not to mention the other meds we got rid of. You are what you eat and we are living proof, thanks to The Diet of Hope lifestyle change.
Quote by Glenn and Georgia Pfleiderer

Lost 52 lbs   Lost 90 lbs   Lost 50 lbs   Lost 50 lbs

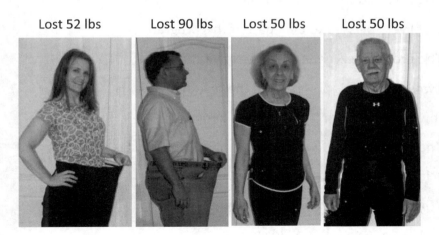

Satisfaction

At the end of our 6 weeks (phase one) program we ask our patients to fill out a questionnaire and rate our program on a scale of one to five; five being excellent.

Of 4,250 patients, 97% gave us a 5 rating, 2.8% a 4 rating and 8 patients rated the program a 3.

Now, 170 physicians or nurse practitioners in Tucson refer patients to us.

Twenty eight local physicians were patients in our program. Twenty three of these physicians have achieved long term success.

Quotes from our Patients
(From a Questionnaire)

- I feel I got another chance in life.
- I feel very blessed to be a part of this program.
- The program exceeded all my expectations.
- I will stay on this program for the rest of my life.
- It works and doesn't cost an arm and a leg.
- The program works because it makes sense; it is medically and scientifically sound.
- I thought I knew it all. Now the light is on.
- This is not a diet, it is a life change.
- I never felt hungry.

Quotes from our Patients (Continued)
(From a Questionnaire)

- The program is easy to follow and affordable.

- My joints don't hurt anymore, the swelling is gone.

- I got my life back.

- Better than any program I have been on.

- This program addresses health not just weight.

- This program deserves more than a five, it is a ten.

CHAPTER 10

LONGEVITY AND CALORIES

Some people eat to live and others live to eat. We all want to live a long, healthy life and die peacefully of old age in our sleep. Multiple diets exist. They all have the same goal: a long and healthy life. There is a common denominator between successful diets. Low fat diets, low carb diets, vegetarian diets, and Mediterranean diets: they all avoid sugar and refined carbohydrates.

A calorie restricted diet is another approach. Roy Walford, a pathology professor at UCLA, wrote a book "The Retardation of Aging and Disease by Dietary Restriction" in 1988. He showed in experiments with mice that severe calorie restrictions can double their lifespan. These experiments were repeated with many animal species and rendered similar results.

Walford was the medical leader of an experiment at the Biosphere near Tucson. Eight scientists lived for two years in the enclosed Biosphere, eating only from what they could produce. It was all plant food. The production of food was less than expected and all eight scientists went on a calorie restricted diet. In addition, the diet was low in protein and fat. They felt miserable and were hungry all the time. While they lost weight, lowered their cholesterol and blood pressure, they eventually needed food from the outside world. Doctor Walford died at age seventy nine from amyotrophic lateral sclerosis (ALS). Further animal studies later showed that calorie restriction accelerates ALS.

Rhesus monkeys are genetically closely related to humans. A 14-year study on rhesus macaques monkeys at the University of Wisconsin-Madison compared two groups of monkeys, one was allowed unlimited monkey chow and the other group was given 30% less of the same food. The calorie-restricted group showed a trend toward reduced death rates and a significant delay in age-related diseases and aging overall.

In contrast to the conclusion reached at the University of Wisconsin-Madison, a similar study performed by the National Institute of Aging (NIA) found no survival benefit with calorie restriction. However, they did not use the same monkey chow. Now the two groups of scientists need to go back to the drawing board and decide what is a healthy diet for monkeys in captivity?

Nathan Pritikin founded the Longevity Center in California in 1975. His mission was to reduce heart disease and prolong a healthy life with a vegetarian diet and exercise. He advocated that only 5 to 10 of calories should come from fat, 10 to 15% from protein and 75 to 85%from carbohydrates. At age 69 he had developed leukemia and committed suicide. Dealing with one issue may create another problem. Data from the Nurses' Health Study showed women, who consumed more fat, including saturated fat, had a lower incidence of breast cancer. In Pritikin's days we did not know much about the good and essential fats (Omega Fats). A diet too low in fat may not be healthy.

How many calories does our body need on a daily basis? While this a simple question, it lacks a straight answer. You can find calculators on the internet. I used four different calculators, and they all suggested I should eat between 2,500 calories to 2,700 calories per day. If I eat more than 1,500 calories I gain weight. Of course, the calculator also tells me at least 60% of my calories should come from carbohydrates.

Alan Keys used conscientious objectors during the war and fed them what he considered a starvation diet of 1,500 calories, mostly in the form of cheap carbohydrates. They all lost weight and felt miserable; they also lost a significant amount of muscle and lean tissue. After the end of the study they all gained their weight back. This was one of the studies that convinced people diets don't work. What Keys missed was that carbohydrates do not provide sufficient nutrition; these poor individuals were actually starving. If they would have received sufficient protein and fat they might have been happy with 1,200 calories.

The average daily calorie consumption in women in 1970 was 1,542 calories; in the year 2,000 it increased by 335 calories to 1,877 calories. The average consumption by men in 1970 was 2,450 calories and increased 168 calories to 2,618 calories. The increase in calories was mostly due to increased carbohydrate consumption, especially sweetened beverages. Certainly, women in 1970 on 1,542 calories were not starving. Maybe that is the adequate amount of calories for women as long as they receive enough protein, fat, vitamins and minerals.

We need to go back to the basics. Our body needs protein, good fats, vitamins, minerals and phytonutrients from vegetables. Carbohydrates are optional. The only effective treatment for obesity is reducing carbohydrates including "healthy whole wheat". Women 40 years ago consumed 1,542 calories per day. They were not starving. They were healthier. On average, I have consumed 1,500 calories per day for the last 15 years, and I exercise an hour a day. I don't feel starved. We should rethink our calorie needs.

Barry Sears promoted his Zone Diet in 1995. His diet was composed of 30% protein, 30% fat and 40% carbohydrates. He calculated the body's protein need based on lean body weight. His diet was promoted heavily on Cardiology Meetings. When I did my calculations my body needed 1,200 calories per day. Many people would consider this a starvation diet, but it is not.

Hjalmar Stevenson did his year-long dietary experiment at a New York hospital eating an Eskimo diet (Fat and meat). His diet consisted of 30% protein and 70% fat. He stayed healthy; however when the investigators tried to reduce his fat intake he developed severe diarrhea. He consumed close to 3,000 calories and did not gain weight. So, like always, when we deal with nutrition there are differing opinions.

Intermittent fasting is becoming popular. A 24 hour fast obviously reduces calorie intake. It also produces a mild state of ketosis indicating that the body metabolism has changed to metabolize fat, therefore causing extra weight loss.

CHAPTER 11

OBESITY

Not all cases of obesity are caused by dietary factors. Genetics play a role. We all have seen women with big hips and small upper bodies, or men with spindly legs and big bellies. Obesity frequently runs in families. Women and men have different fat distribution, presumably related to our sex hormones. There is the famous report of a 12 year old girl burning her hand. She was treated with a skin transplant from her abdomen. At age twenty-eight, when she grew quite obese, her hand ballooned with fat, requiring liposuction. This suggests that local factors in fat cells are involved in fat accumulation.

The present obesity epidemic is clearly related to the excessive consumption of carbohydrates. The recommendation from our government (USDA) and medical societies to consume 60% of our calories from carbohydrates is not only wrong, but it is a part of the obesity problem.

The Center for Medicare and Medicaid has recently released new guidelines for the treatment of obesity. Physicians can now treat obesity as a serious medical problem. This is a major reversal of previous policies. The American Medical Association has declared that obesity is a disease. This will place pressure on insurance companies to pay for the treatment of obesity. Physicians are urged to address obesity at every patient's visit. Moreover, electronic medical records now require documentation of a patient's body mass index (BMI). A BMI is a number derived from dividing a person's weight by their height squared in the metric system. A BMI of 20 to 25 is considered normal; a BMI of 25 to 30 indicates overweight, and above 30 indicates obesity. The numbers were developed by the insurance industry. For example, if one's BMI is above 45, then according to insurance statistics, life expectancy will be shortened by at least 15 years.

Obesity rates are soaring; in the U.S. childhood obesity has more than doubled in the last 30 years and has tripled in adolescents. Non-Hispanic blacks have the highest age adjusted rates of obesity (49.5%) compared with Mexican Americans (39.4%). Worldwide obesity has nearly doubled since 1980. So it is not just a U.S. problem. This year Mexico's population has become overall heavier than the U.S. population. At least the Mexican government responded to the epidemic of obesity with a soda tax and taxes on certain snacks.

In addition, First Lady Michelle Obama is trying to address childhood obesity. She is being "out-foxed" by the food industry. French fries are now considered vegetables.

Causes for the obesity epidemic are multiple. The National Institute of Health (NIH) states the obvious: overweight and obesity happen over time when you take in more calories than you use. The real question is why do we eat more than we need? Later in the book, we will discuss how the old theory of "a calorie is a calorie" doesn't hold up any more. Our body responds to carbohydrates differently than to protein and fat. Carbohydrates make you fat, fat doesn't make you fat. Any farmer taking care of cows and pigs knows the secret of fattening animals is feeding them corn and soy. We know that women over the last 30 years increased their daily calorie intake by 335 calories and men by 168 calories. Almost all of these extra calories came from carbohydrates.

Our government still insists that 60% of our calories should come from carbohydrates.

Our eating behavior and our food environment have changed dramatically over the last 40 years. We don't have to cook anymore. Fast food restaurants are at every corner, providing us with inexpensive food thanks to the subsidies from our government. This fast food is unhealthy because it is full of sugar and fat, produced in factories. Some of the fat in fast food is *trans* fat, well known to cause heart disease. Supersizing a meal is another trick of the food industry to make consumers believe they got a good deal. The food industry still makes money, again because of the subsidies they receive from the government. In other words, taxpayers cover the cost. The food is tasty for most people, and addictive for some. The food industry knows how to mix sugar, fat, salt and texture that the food becomes a treat for our pleasure center, the nucleus accumbens. The result is that we want more.

What is more, fast food and sodas are advertised incessantly. Young children are especially easy prey. Advertising works.

The lack of exercise is frequently quoted as an explanation for obesity. I explain my position in the chapter on exercise. I don't believe it plays a major role. The overconsumption of cheap refined carbohydrates is the true culprit.

Obesity is associated with a higher incidence of diabetes, high blood pressure, heart disease, osteoarthritis, sleep apnea, cancer, metabolic syndrome and depression.

Weight Gain Post-Hysterectomy

I was always surprised that most American women gained weight after a hysterectomy. To my knowledge, the uterus doesn't produce any significant hormones. Then I discovered that most surgeons in this country remove the ovaries at the same time. Ovaries produce estrogen. Estrogen plays a role in fat metabolism. Estrogen influences a hormone called lipoprotein lipase (LPL). If LPL is attached to a fat cell it will open channels that facilitate the entry of fat into fat cells. Estrogen inhibits LPL, it prevents fat accumulation. After an ovarectomy, estrogen levels fall and LPL remains uninhibited. Thus, fat accumulation occurs. Gaining weight after an ovarectomy is a hormonal problem, not a matter of willpower.

Growth Hormone (HGH) is produced in the anterior pituitary gland located at the base of the brain. The major role is to stimulate liver and other tissues to secret insulin like growth factor (IGF-1). The New England Journal reported in 1990 a study of 12 elderly men who had low growth hormone levels and were injected with growth hormone for 6 months. They lost 14.1% of fat tissue, gained 8.8% of lean body mass and increased bone density. Several other studies since then have confirmed the results. It is a forbidden substance in athletes. Growth hormone has been hailed as an anti-aging drug that also combats obesity. However, the potential side effects are substantial: diabetes, hypertension, worsening of heart disease and possibly cancer promotion, especially prostate cancer.

Testosterone, considered a male hormone, is also present in women. Results from the European Male Aging Study found that obesity is a major cause of low testosterone levels. Low levels of testosterone are found in 75% of men of all ages with a BMI greater 40. Decreases in testosterone seen in men as they get older might be related to gradual weight gain over many years. Testosterone levels even in older men can become normal with weight loss (EUR J Endocrinal 2013; 168). Previously it was assumed that the decrease in testosterone levels seen in older men was due to age, but the age-related study showed that the drop in testosterone is actually due to weight gain. So it is not a low testosterone level that makes people gain weight. Rather, obesity interferes with our hormone production, although the reason is unknown. This study should be a major enforcer for people to lose weight.

Adiponectin is a recently (1996) discovered hormone produced exclusively by our fat tissue. Levels of adiponectin are inversely related with body fat percentage in adults. The more fat we have, the less adiponectin is produced. Adiponectin has a wide range of functions: It decreases gluconeogenesis (the production of glucose from protein), improves insulin resistance, clears triglycerides, improves endothelial function, helps weight loss. Low levels of adiponectin are an independent risk factor for diabetes and the metabolic syndrome.

Leptin is another hormone produced in our fat tissue. At one time leptin was thought to be the answer to obesity. The production of leptin parallels the amount of fat we have. It regulates body weight. Leptin stimulates part of our hypothalamus that control feeding behavior, hunger and energy expenditure. Unfortunately high levels of insulin block the leptin effect on the brain. Obesity is frequently associated with high insulin levels.

Ghrelin is a hormone produced mostly in the stomach; it is called the hunger hormone. It is elevated before a meal. Moreover, it is responsible for the growling noises in our stomach when we are hungry. After a meal ghrelin blood levels decrease. Ghrelin is an appetite inducer and affects feeding behavior. Ghrelin levels are lower in obese person compared to lean people, which would suggest it does not contribute to obesity, except in the rare disease called Prader-Willi syndrome. These patients produce excessive amounts of ghrelin and therefore get hungrier and eat more.

A hormone peptide YY (PYY) is produced in the small intestine. When food reaches the stomach ghrelin production lowers, and we are no longer hungry. The food has to reach the small intestines which will take at least 15 minutes before PPY is produced that signals satiety.

CHAPTER 12

EXERCISE AND OBESITY

For the obese patient, exercise to lose weight is wishful thinking. Do the math: light exercise, such as walking and gardening, burns an average of 4 calories per minute (240 calories per hour). Moderate exercise, such as brisk walking, tennis and modest hiking, burns 6 calories per minute (360 calories per hour). Heavy exercise, such as jogging, vigorous hiking, racquet ball and cross country skiing, burn an average 10 calories per minute (600 calories per hour).

One pound of body fat contains 3,500 calories.

On average, to lose one pound of fat a person must exercise 1 hour per day, for 10 days and not increase the amount of food they consume. So, after exercising for 10 days, a person weighing 300 pounds will weigh 299 pounds. How discouraging! However, this same person can accomplish the same weight loss by not eating a bagel for breakfast. Portion control and avoiding fattening carbohydrates should be the initial treatment for obesity. This approach is far more effective. With the Diet of Hope, this person can expect to lose 20 to 30 pounds in 6 weeks.

Extremely obese patients generally cannot or do not exercise. They simply do not have the energy. Their bodies are in a fat storing mode, their insulin levels are high, and they have no access to their stored fat; therefore, they lack energy. Once their metabolism switches to a fat consuming mode, they feel more energetic and actually feel like exercising.

Exercise is far more helpful in maintaining weight. We can have the bagel after an hour of exercise. Though we won't lose weight, we will maintain our weight.

We all know we can work up an appetite with exercise. The food industry knows this too. For this reason, it is not uncommon to find food places next to a gym, ready to reward us for our efforts.

The more muscles we have, the more calories we burn. When we measure the basal metabolism of our obese patients who carry an extra 100 pounds, and therefore have more muscle, their metabolism is usually slightly above normal. Oftentimes these patients are surprised because they assumed they were suffering from slow metabolism.

Increasing muscles through weight lifting stimulates our metabolism. However, the effects are small. If we replace 5 pounds of fat with 5 pounds of muscle through weightlifting our metabolism increases only by 24 calories a day, the calories of four potato chips(Gary Taubes).

If we weigh ourselves before we go to bed and again early in the morning, we will discover that most weight loss occurs at night while we asleep. The better and deeper the sleep, the more weight loss occurs. It is thought during a good sleep the body releases growth hormone. Growth hormone stimulates cell regeneration and growth and helps build muscle mass. This activity stimulates the metabolism. Good sleep lowers cortisol levels. High cortisol levels leads to a lower metabolism. Lack of sleep lowers leptin and increases ghrelin, which results in an increase of appetite. Leptin is a hormone released by our fat cells. Leptin sends a satiety signal to the brain. Ghrelin produced by the stomach stimulates hunger. So lower Leptin levels signal to the brain that we need more energy, we have to eat; high Ghrelin levels make us hungry. A good night sleep is important for us. Sleep deprivation can cause weight gain.

The health club industry has over 10,000 clubs in the US with over 50 million members, with an annual income of over 20 billion dollars. This industry has grown dramatically over the last 40 years. Some cynics say the growth of health clubs has paralleled the epidemic of obesity. Again, exercise alone for the treatment of obesity, in my opinion, is not very effective. However, exercise is helpful for weight maintenance.

My wife and I are strong believers in exercise; we have sponsored a 10 kilometer race (Cinco de Mayo race in Tucson) for the last 15 years. We play tennis three times a week, we run, we hike, and we enjoy bicycle tours. During our honeymoon we climbed Kilimanjaro in Africa.

Benefits of Exercise:

1. Improves chances to live longer and healthier
2. Protects against developing heart disease, lowers blood pressure and cholesterol
3. Helps prevent adult onset of diabetes
4. Helps prevent arthritis
5. Helps prevent osteoporosis
6. Reduces the risk of falling in older patients
7. Relieves symptoms of depression and anxiety
8. Helps to maintain healthy weight
9. Helps keep you agile

CHAPTER 13

THE LAW OF THERMODYNAMICS

Energy is neither created nor destroyed, but can only change from one form to another. Those who consume more calories than they expend in energy will gain weight. While this law is correct, it does not explain what makes us eat more and why our bodies like to store fat. We can accuse our poor patients of eating excessively or not exercising enough. While this is true, it offers little explanation. We need to ask the questions: What does the body do with the food we eat? How do we digest certain food? What is the hormonal response to food? What causes fat storage? How does our brain respond to different food?

We can come up with many excuses for our patients: we live in a toxic food environment, too many fast food restaurants tempt us with ever-increasing portions, we don't cook anymore, we don't exercise enough, we are under the influence of the clever food industry, our government and the medical societies are of no help, we don't eat enough protein or fat, and we eat too many carbohydrates. Why does our body love carbohydrates? Why do we store carbohydrates as fat? Here is where our hormones play an important role.

The master hormone is insulin. Its main task is to keep our sugar level as close to normal as possible. The carbohydrates we eat end up as sugar in our blood stream. Insulin takes care of the glucose and fructose goes directly to the liver. Glucose can be stored as glycogen in our muscles and liver. The storage amount is limited, excessive sugar gets stored as fat. So, insulin is a storage hormone. It is the controller of our fat tissue. As long as insulin levels are elevated, no fat can be released. Therefore, carbohydrates we eat enter a one way street to our fat tissue. As long as insulin levels are elevated, the body has no access to the food recently consumed. For this reason, we may feel tired two to three hours after we eat. It is as if we are out of gasoline and need to eat again.

While this is a simplified explanation, it effectively explains our behavior. Clearly, fat doesn't make us overweight, it is the carbohydrates we consume that make us fat. For example, feedlots for cows use sweet corn to fatten their animals.

So, if we want to encourage our body to change from a fat storage mode, to a fat consuming mode, we need to reduce our insulin levels. We have learned that excessive fructose consumption can lead to liver insulin resistance raising our insulin levels. What is more, after excessive prolonged glucose consumption, our muscles become insulin resistant, again more insulin is needed to process glucose. Unfortunately, fat tissue rarely becomes insulin resistant. Insulin resistance has several consequences. Higher insulin levels maintain the body in the fat storage mode. Moreover, higher insulin levels stimulate cholesterol production in the liver. Insulin also affects the kidneys by stimulating salt and water retention, which can increase blood pressure. Lastly, higher insulin levels are known to stimulate cancer growth.

CHAPTER 14

CARBOHYDRATES, SACCHARIDES OR SUGARS

Carbohydrates are one of the three macronutrients (along with proteins and fats). Carbohydrates supply energy (calories). The human body *can* function without carbohydrates. Humans are able to obtain 100% of their energy requirements from proteins and fat.

The 2010 Dietary Guidelines for Americans (USDA) call for moderate to high carbohydrate consumption. The guidelines suggest that a "so-called" balanced diet should include six, one-ounce servings of a grain food each day; it is suggested that at least half of these servings derive from whole grain sources and the rest from enriched (refined) grains.

Types of Carbohydrates:

Monosaccharides *(sugars that contain one molecule)*:

- Glucose
- Fructose
- Galactose

Disaccharides *(two sugar molecules are combined)*:

- Sucrose or table sugar is formed of glucose and fructose; sucrose is synthetized only by plants.
- High fructose corn syrup is 55% fructose and 45% glucose made from corn.
- Lactose or milk sugar is a combination of galactose and glucose.
- Maltose consists of two units of glucose in beer.

Polysaccharides *(multiple sugar molecules are combined)*:

- Glycogen is the storage form of glucose in muscle and liver.
- Every gram of glycogen is stored with three grams of water.
- We can store a total of 1,200 calories as glycogen in our muscles and liver.
- Cellulose is the major form of fiber in our diet from vegetables, fruits and nuts.
- Starches such as bread, rice and potatoes contain only glucose, no fructose.

SUCROSE (Table Sugar)

The only sugar available 150 years ago was sugar derived from sugar cane, originally introduced from Asia. This sugar was relatively expensive. My great, great grandmother kept sugar cubes in a silver box. Then sugar beet became available around 1870. It was relatively cheap and that's when sugar consumption started to rise. In 1960 the average sugar consumption was 120 pounds per person per year. Then, in the 1970's high fructose corn syrup was introduced. It was the cheapest sugar because of the subsidies our government granted to the corn industry. Now, the average sugar consumption is at least 150 pounds per person, per year. The government pays 20 billion dollars a year to subsidize corn and soy production.

Why is Sugar Toxic?

In his book, Fat Chance, Dr. Robert Lustig argues that sugar is toxic to the body.

The human body has never been exposed to excessive amounts of sugar before. The average adult person carries five liters of blood. Those five liters contain one teaspoon of glucose, reflecting a normal blood sugar level of 65 to 99 mg/dl or roughly 4 to 5 grams of glucose. A 12 ounce can of Coca-Cola has 39 grams of sugar or at least 8 teaspoons of sugar. Insulin is our hormone that defends us against fluctuations of blood sugar. Insulin opens channels that allow glucose to enter muscles, liver and other organ systems. Insulin converts excessive sugar to fat and stores it in our fat tissue.

To measure the challenge to the insulin system we use an index called glycemic index. It measures the two hour blood sugar response to a given load of 50 grams of a food. Glucose is the standard and has a glycemic index of 100. Unfortunately, there is an alternate method that uses white bread as the standard index of 100. The more refined food is the quicker and higher the sugar rises. In the original system, the glycemic index of white bread was 69 and whole wheat bread was 72, while table sugar (sucrose) was 59. Table sugar consists of glucose and fructose. Fructose has a glycemic index of 20. Other examples of glycemic index are baked potato 98, instant rice 91, and cornflake cereal 80. Fat and protein have a glycemic index of 0 (Source: *Wheat Belly*)

A continuous bombardment of our body with high glycemic food, especially glucose, stresses the insulin capability. Muscles and liver cannot cope with the massive influx of glucose and become insulin resistant. This is the very early stage of the metabolic syndrome, and can lead to diabetes. However, our fat tissue is the last to become insulin resistant, fat accumulation continues on a high carbohydrate diet.

Fructose

Sucrose is 50% glucose and 50% fructose. High fructose corn syrup is 45% glucose and 55% fructose, not much of a difference. Fructose consumption has increased fivefold over the last century. Twenty-five percent of calories we consume come from sugars. Fruits are now available all year long, in the past they were available only during harvest time. Most fruits are hybrids designed to be very sweet. Sweetness is related to fructose; fructose is much sweeter than glucose. Fructose does not stimulate insulin release and raises blood sugar levels very little. In the past, the Diabetic Association felt that fructose would be ideal for diabetics. But, fructose might be worse than glucose. Fructose moves from the gut directly to the liver. The liver is the primary site for fructose metabolism. The liver has only a limited capacity to process fructose (Source: Robert H. Lustig).

Fructose cannot be converted into glycogen, the storage form of glucose. Fructose metabolism requires energy; if the energy is exhausted then fructose can be changed to uric acid, which can cause gout. Most of the fructose reaching the liver is converted to fat, causing a fatty liver, which can eventually progress to liver cirrhosis. Nonalcoholic, fatty liver cirrhosis is now the third most common cause for the need of liver transplants. Latinos have a high incidence of diabetes and nonalcoholic fatty liver. Nineteen percent of Latinos have a genetic defect that makes them highly sensitive to fructose.

Prolonged excessive fructose consumption causes liver insulin resistance, which leads to hyper insulinemia. Hyper insulinemia frequently leads to excessive body fat storage. High insulin levels promote cancer growth.

Fructose does not produce satiety; rather it stimulates reward centers in our brain that tempt us to eat more of the same. The capacity of the liver to metabolize fructose is thought to be 50 grams.

A recent study in the Journal of American Medical Association (JAMA, February 2014) found that high sugar consumption doubles the chance of dying from heart disease.

CHAPTER 15

DIABETES

Diabetes is preventable and often reversible! Twenty-Six million Americans are diabetic; seven million Americans don't know that they are diabetic. They all have an A1C of 6.5% or higher. Seventy-nine million Americans are prediabetic, with an A1C from 5.7% to 6.4%. People ages 65 or older have a 26.9% higher incidence of diabetes than younger adults. Seventy percent of diabetics have neurological problems such as neuropathies. Risks of heart disease and strokes quadruple. Risk of dementia doubles (Diabetes Type 3). Diabetes is the leading cause for blindness and renal failure. Sixty percent of lower leg amputations occur in diabetics.

The cost of treatment of diabetes in 2007 was 174 billion dollars, by now it is probably above 200 billion dollars (Source: American Diabetic Association).

The medical profession is helpless in the treatment of this dreadful disease. We have more and more expensive new medications. We have no data on their long term effect or side effects. Medications are not a cure. As my diabetic mother–in-law often complained to me, "I have followed all the recommendations from my doctors, I took all my medications faithfully including insulin and what happened, my kidneys are failing, my legs needed amputations. What kind of treatment is this?"

Dietitians still teach diabetic patients to eat 50-60 grams of carbohydrates with each meal; this recommendation is based on an old metabolic study from 40 years ago. Further discussion on this topic may be found in the chapter on Ketones. Our body can function well without eating carbohydrates.

For example, in the past, Eskimos had no access to carbohydrates. It is not a coincidence that they had no diabetes or heart disease. How did their brain function without carbohydrates? Our liver can produce glucose from protein. What is more, the brain also functions well with ketones.

The pharmaceutical industry controls the treatment of diabetes. They have convinced the general population that diets do not work in the treatment of diabetes. Their answer to diabetes is medications. If a patient sees a doctor and their blood sugar is elevated, they are diagnosed with diabetes. Oftentimes, the doctor pays lip service to diets and then prescribes a pill. The most commonly prescribed pills are called sulfonylureas; they force the pancreas to make more insulin. Sulfonylureas have been implicated in several studies, such as the Accord Study, to increase mortality possibly related to intermittent hypoglycemia. The other problem with sulfonylureas is that they do not affect the underlying problem. They overstress the pancreas, the pancreas eventually gives up and the patient has to go on insulin.

Type 2 Diabetes is related to what we eat! The epidemic of diabetes and obesity is directly related to a marked increase of carbohydrate consumption. While newer diabetic medications are superior to older medications, they have not stood the test of time and they are tremendously expensive. A study with 10,000 diabetic patients showed that control of blood sugar with medications such as insulin and sulfonylureas increased the death rate of the patients that reached an A1C level below 7 (Source: *Accord Study*). The excessive death rate was probably related to hypoglycemic episodes. So, now we are told not to aim at normal A1C levels. We know elevated A1C levels directly correlate with the complications of diabetes. Only carbohydrate restricted diets are able to normalize elevated A1C levels without complications.

Our government is helpless against the power of food and pharmaceutical industries. They are important and influential constituents. Plus, our government supports the sugar, corn and wheat industry with massive amounts of subsidies through the Farm Bill.

The suggestion that we should all eat 60% of our calories from carbohydrates is suitable for somebody who is slim and exercises a lot. However, these individuals are becoming a small minority. To tell a diabetic or an obese person to consume 60% of their calories from carbohydrates, even if they are complex carbohydrates, is like promoting obesity and diabetes. Whole wheat is considered to be a complex carbohydrate, but in our body it acts like a simple carbohydrate raising our glucose level very fast and high. While it has more nutrition than refined bread, such nutrition may be obtained from another food that does not raise blood sugar.

Remember how our body handles carbohydrates. The body metabolizes protein and fat differently from carbohydrates. Carbohydrates end up in our blood stream as glucose (the body treats potatoes, rice, whole wheat or sugar the same way).The faster the glucose from the food rises, the more insulin will be released from the pancreas.

The task for insulin is to maintain a normal blood sugar level. As we discussed in a previous chapter, there is only one teaspoon of sugar in our five liters of blood. When we introduce a load of sugar into our system, Insulin opens multiple channels in our muscles, liver and other organ systems to dispose of the glucose. This works well if it happens occasionally. However, if high glucose levels occur on a regular basis, the muscle and liver eventually become reluctant to accept this high glucose load, and insulin resistance develops. This becomes the very early stage of diabetes. The pancreas responds with an increased production of insulin, forcing the body to accept the glucose load. Prolonged over-production of insulin eventually exhausts the pancreas and true diabetes develops.

One of the solutions for the body is to turn sugar into fat and store it in our fat tissue. This is another task for insulin. So, the prime task for insulin is to control our blood sugar. As long as insulin is elevated, fat will be produced from glucose and send to our fat cells. As a result, fat cannot be released. Essentially, glucose enters a one way street from the blood stream to our fat tissue. Obesity is the end result.

Why is it so important to have a normal blood sugar? Glucose has the tendency to bind with protein anywhere in the body and makes this protein nonfunctional. We call this glucose-protein connections advanced glycation end products (AGES). One of this advanced glycation end products is Hemoglobin A1C. The higher the A1C the more damage is done to the protein in our hemoglobin. Luckily, we replace our red cells every two to three months. This is how we can estimate our blood sugar level over the preceding months. Unfortunately, not all protein is replaced every two to three months and permanent damage can occur such as peripheral neuropathy, kidney and eye damage. It is important to remember those damages can already occur at the "so called" prediabetic stage. Unfortunately, treatment with the medications available cause more harm than good.

The best treatment for this problem is diet, especially the Diet of Hope. Physicians and the public have been reluctant to accept the idea that diabetes can be reversed and prevented through a diet change.

There is a strong belief, based on past experiences that diets do not work in the long run. We beg to differ. We now have data with over 1,000 diabetic patients that have learned the importance of making changes in their eating habits, giving them more control to manage their diabetes or prediabetes. Simply avoiding foods that cause or worsen diabetes is a huge incentive for patient because they learn what foods drives up blood sugar. We even have strong data indicating that patients on insulin for years may be able to stop insulin.

Another common argument against reversal or prevention of diabetes is: my mother and my sister are diabetic, so I will be a diabetic. Wrong again. While there a genetic precondition occurs, the genes have to be activated by what we eat. My wife's family history is a clear example of this. Her mother died from diabetes with kidney failure, with both her lower legs amputated. Another of my wife's uncles is blind from diabetes, two uncles died from diabetes and seven siblings are diabetic. However, my wife has no inkling of diabetes. We have been following our Diet of Hope for the last 15 years.

A unique case of widespread diabetes exists amongst the Pima Indians, a tribe living in the Gila River area near Phoenix. Eighty percent of the Pima Indians are diabetic at age thirty. The Pima Indians were introduced to white flour, sugar, dried fruits and sodas by our "benevolent" government, after their water supply was shut off for irrigation and they were starving. The majority of Pima Indians are markedly overweight because they got hooked on carbohydrates. The same genetically equal people living in Mexico in the Sierra Madre Mountains have an incidence of diabetes of 4%; their average weight is 145 pounds. So, while diabetic genes are important, they have to be activated by what we eat. Again, I have to emphasize that diabetes can be prevented and can frequently be reversed.

Eating 6 to 11 servings of bread, pasta, cereal and rice, as the food pyramid suggests, is a terrible suggestion. We call the food pyramid evil. The new food plate is an improvement but still overemphasizes grains. Obese and diabetic patients, should not follow those suggestions. What is more, I disagree with the idea that we should eat a lot of fruits and vegetables. Non-starchy vegetables can be consumed ad libitum. Fruits are a different story. They should be consumed in limited quantities. Today's fruits are not like our grandparents' fruits, fruits today are all hybrids specifically created to be extra sweet with a lot of fructose. We discussed the problem with fructose in a previous chapter. Doctor Bernstein, a Type 1 diabetic at age eighty (and healthy) told us in a meeting of the Obesity Society that he had not eaten fruits in 40 years because fruits made it difficult to control his blood sugar. He stated, "The value of fruits is overrated." Having fruits year round is new in our history. Fruits were only available at harvest time in the past. Our bodies have not had enough time to adjust to daily fruit consumption.

Cost of Medications in Dollars

(Prices in Tucson Arizona as of January 2014)

Insulins

	Pharmacy A	Pharmacy B	
Humalog vial	216.99	112.20	70/30
Novolog vial	214.99	205.99	
Humalog disposable pen	537.99	385.20	
Novolog Flex pen	425.99	395.99	
Vial of Lantus	225.99	231.99	
Solostar Lantus	391.99	359.99	
Vial of Levemir	289.99	235.99	
Levemir Flexpen	345.99	384.99	
Humulin R U-500	1,102.00	1,000.00	
Humulin N 100	91.98	112.20	

Monthly Cost

Pramlintide 120mg	1,404.99	2,095.00
Byetta 10 mcg bid	450.99	374.99
Victoza 1.8	375.99	423.99
Januvia	320.99	323.99

Weight Loss Medication

Belviq 10mg #30	127.99	125.49
Qsymia #30	159.99	187.99

CHAPTER 16

KETONES

What are ketones? Fat is stored in our fat cells as triglycerides. Three fatty acids are connected to glycerol molecule. When triglycerides leave a fat cell they are broken down in fatty acids and glycerol. Glycerol can be converted to sugar. Our liver can split fatty acid into ketones. Three ketones are created: acetacetic acid, beta-hydroxybutyric acid and acetones. Beta-hydroxybutiric acid and aceteacedic acid can cross the blood brain barrier and provide the brain with energy. Acetone can be eliminated by the kidneys and lungs (actually helping us to lose calories).

Ketosis is a metabolic state in our body, where the body switches from a pure sugar energy processing mode to utilizing fat as the main energy provider. All of us change to that mode if we don't eat for 12 hours. The body depletes the sugar reserves which are limited and turns to fat as energy source. The maximal storage capacity for carbohydrates is 1,200 calories derived from glycogen in muscles and liver. A marathon runner will hit the wall at 20 miles of running. His body is out of glycogen and has to switch to fatty acids and ketones.

Certainly most of us have fat energy supplies that can last for weeks or longer. Fasting, prolonged exercise, low carbohydrate diets produce a mild state of ketosis.

Benign ketosis should not be confused with diabetic ketoacidosis; a severe complication in diabetics who can no longer process glucose due to lack of insulin.

If we want to lose weight and get rid of our excessive fat stores then we need to mobilize our fat. Fat has to leave the fat cells, has to travel to our liver and our liver changes fatty acids into ketones. Ketones are the markers that tell us our body has switched from sugar to fat as its preferred energy provider. So, ketones in our blood are desirable.

We get frustrated if one of our successful patients consults a diabetic dietitian and is told they have to eat at least 50 grams of carbohydrates with each meal. This recommendation dates back to a study 40 years ago where the sugar consumption of the brain was measured. This study showed that our brain uses 120 grams to 140 grams of sugar over a period of 24 hours. However, what the study missed is that if sugar is the only energy provider available the brain will use it exclusively. If ketones are available, our brain will use ketones too. (Source: *Basic Neurochemistry,* 6th edition Siegel et al: Lippincott; 1999). A ketogenic diet (low carbohydrate diet) was developed for children with seizures who were unresponsive to medications. Ketones calmed the brain and seizures cleared. Such evidence suggests that ketones are beneficial for the brain.

Some cells in our body, including parts of our brain, can use only glucose. Our liver is perfectly capable of creating glucose from protein. Most diabetics are aware of sugar production by the liver. They go to bed with a normal blood sugar, eat nothing all night, but the blood sugar is elevated in the morning. Their liver created glucose from protein. We use Metformin to block the liver from making glucose from protein. Recommending that a diabetic eat sugar is condemning them to a state of permanent diabetes and all its complications.

CHAPTER 17

ADDICTION

The Webster's Dictionary definition of "addiction" is:

> *A strong harmful need to regularly have something or do something, a compulsive physiological need for and use of a habit forming substance, characterized by tolerance and by well-defined physiological symptoms upon withdrawal.*

Can food be addictive? The answer is: definitely, yes! A patient of ours, a recovered heroin addict, came back after the first week on our program and told us when he stopped eating sugar and refined carbohydrates he became nauseated, developed diarrhea, and started to sweat. For him the withdrawal from carbohydrates was almost as bad as the withdrawal from heroin.

Several years ago, I was at a medical meeting. Next door the food industry also had a meeting. I was curious and listened to one presentation. A new food was created with a mix of fat, sugar and salt; it was crunchy. It was tested on 10 volunteers with a functional MRI. The test showed that a small area in the midbrain was activated, which is considered a pleasure center. The experts expected that this food would sell very well. This is an example of how the food industry manipulates us.

A new weight loss medication Ribonabant first came on the market in Europe. It was very effective in producing weight loss. However, it was withdrawn from the market when some patients became suicidal. It blocked the pleasure center too effectively.

The pleasure center is called Nucleus Accumbens, a structure in the basal forebrain. It is the key structure of the brain responsible for reward, motivation and addiction. Sugar and carbohydrates stimulate this center through the neurotransmitter dopamine the same way as addictive drugs do. Fat is not stimulatory, however some proteins are. One is gluten, the main protein in wheat. During digestion of gluten, polypeptides are released that can penetrate the blood brain barrier and create an opium like effect on the brain. This stimulates our pleasure center, which could be a possible cause of food addiction (Source: *Wheat Belly*). The action of these polypeptides can be prevented with opiate-blocking drugs naloxone and naltrexone.

CHAPTER 18

HISTORY OF THE LOW FAT DIET

After world war two, a significant increase in heart disease occurred. Heart attacks frequently affected middle age men without warning. Congressmen and senators were not spared. President Eisenhower had a heart attack in 1955. Doctor Paul Dudley White became his cardiologist. Dr. Dudley noted that before 1930 he rarely if ever saw a heart attack patient, but after the war it appeared an epidemic of heart disease was occurring. The medical community was searching for answers. Some of the epidemic was related to increased longevity, people didn't die from infectious diseases any more since the discovery of antibiotics. But this still did not fully explain the epidemic.

Several scientific studies from the 1940 have revealed a correlation between very high levels of cholesterol and coronary artery disease. Cholesterol became the suspect.

After the war, Ancel Keys a scientist from the University of Minnesota received a yearly $100,000 grant to study diets in different countries. Some early research data suggested that a high intake of fat may raise cholesterol levels. Keys had access to nutrition patterns of 22 countries. He picked only seven countries where he could demonstrate a correlation between saturated fat consumption and higher cholesterol levels, which presumably increase the risk of heart attacks. In the other 15 countries he could not show that correlation. So he had to exclude countries like France, Holland, Switzerland.

A study like this would not be given any scientific merit today. Also in those days only total cholesterol could be measured, the concept of good and bad cholesterol was not available yet. Later studies showed that saturated fat raises the good and the bad cholesterol and therefore, does not increase the risk of heart disease.

Keyes recruited many followers to his hypothesis. Especially scientists from the nutrition departments of the east coast universities such as Harvard and Yale, which became believers of this concept.

Saturated fat and cholesterol were frequently lumped together because food with high saturated fat generally also had high cholesterol levels. However, Keys' own studies showed no correlation between cholesterol intake and cholesterol blood levels. His statement in 1977, "We have known all along that cholesterol in diets does not matter at all except in rabbits." Rabbit cholesterol blood levels can raise 3,000 fold with feeding of cholesterol. Human serum cholesterol levels are essentially independent of the cholesterol intake with the whole range of human diets.

In spite of his statements, dietary cholesterol was singled out as the main culprit in producing heart disease. All food containing cholesterol such as eggs, butter, shrimp and milk were essentially treated as poison. Margarine (*trans* fat), which was the real poison, replaced butter. Polyunsaturated fats such as vegetable oils were recommended initially, but later were found to possibly aggravate or produce cancer.

The diet heart hypothesis became the gospel, then a religion and later a dogma. The medical profession became totally convinced that fat and cholesterol intake was a major risk factor for heart disease and cancer. The hypothesis claimed there was a direct correlation between heart disease and the consumption of saturated fat and cholesterol.

In 1977, the US Senate Select Committee on Nutrition and Human Needs chaired by George McGovern put the diet heart hypothesis on the national agenda with publication on the dietary goals in the United States. McGovern stated that too much fat, too much sugar or too much salt can be, and are directly linked to heart disease, cancer, obesity and stroke. The sugar industry made sure fat was singled out as the main culprit.

The Lipid Research Council Study (LRC) showed that a drug (Cholestyramine) lowered cholesterol and reduced the incidence of heart disease. This was enough evidence for the lead researchers to proclaim that lowering cholesterol with diets will reduce heart disease the same way. So, the assumption was that if lowering cholesterol with medications lowered the risk of heart disease, then lowering cholesterol with diets would render the same result. Unfortunately, manipulations of diets are far more complicated than taking a pill.

No study with diets was done, however it became a belief system. No serious scientific diet study ever conducted proved the diet heart hypothesis.

However, studies contradicting the diet heart hypothesis appeared. The most prominent was the Lyon Heart Study. Six hundred patients who had experienced a heart attack were equally divided to follow the American Heart Association diet or a French Mediterranean diet. The study had to be stopped early. There was a 70% higher mortality rate in the group using the American Heart Association diet.

A one billion dollar study *The Women's Health Initiative* study was supposed to settle the question about low fat diets, the importance of fiber, exercise, and hormone replacement for women. Forty nine thousand women were enrolled. Twenty three thousand women were chosen to go on low fat diet, a diet high in fiber, they were encouraged to exercise and received frequent counseling. The control group was left to their own devices.

The expected result was that the intensively treated group would have a significantly lower rate of heart disease, cancer, diabetes, and obesity. Surprisingly, there was no significant difference between both groups at the end of the eight year study.

If we lower one major food group in our diet, such as fat, we need to increase consumption of another food group such as carbohydrates because protein intake cannot be raised significantly. So it was suggested that all we needed to eat was more carbohydrates. The American Heart Association certified hundreds of carbohydrates (all processed food) as heart healthy. Then, along came the food pyramid, which I refer to as the "Evil Food Pyramid." The Evil Food Pyramid recommended that everyone eat 6 to 11 servings of bread, pasta, cereals and rice on a daily basis. In my opinion, there is a direct relationship between these recommendations and the epidemic of obesity and diabetes in our country.

CHAPTER 19

CIGARETTES: THE MISSING LINK

It is tempting to speculate that a high fat diet was never the culprit of the epidemic of heart disease at the end of World War II. During the war, high fat diets were not available for most populations in the world; so why was high fat consumption blamed for the epidemic of heart disease after the war?

Cigarettes were one of the few pleasures that American GI's could enjoy regardless of where they were. There was nothing more relaxing than a cigarette during moments of respite before returning to the battle.

In 1941, U.S. president Franklin D. Roosevelt made tobacco a protected crop. Cigarettes were included in the daily food rations for GI's. Tobacco companies sent millions of free cigarettes to the troops. The U.S. Army set up a series of camps in France each named after a popular American cigarette such as Lucky Strike, Chesterfield, and Old Gold.

Essentially, the government hooked everybody on cigarettes. It was estimated that in 1949, 90% of the adult male population smoked. Even doctors were advertising that cigarettes might help patients with asthma.

Starting in 1955, questions were raised that cigarette smoke may cause lung disease. In 1956, the American Heart Association issued a statement on smoking and cardiovascular disease. This statement indicated that the evidence available at that time was not sufficiently conclusive on the relationship between smoking and increased death rates from coronary heart disease.

- In 1957, the surgeon general declared a link between smoking and lung cancer.
- In 1963, the FDA expressed its interpretation that tobacco did not qualify for a hazardous substance.
- In 1964, the American Medical Association accepted a $10 million grant from the tobacco industry to conduct tobacco research. The association promised not to make a statement on tobacco until the 10 year study was finished.
- In 1973, Arizona became the first state to pass a law restricting smoking in some public places like elevators, libraries, concert halls and buses.
- In 1973, Billie Jean won the battle of the sexes in tennis against Bobby Riggs. She was promoting Virginia Slims, the cigarette for women.
- In 1988, the surgeon general declared cigarettes were addictive. Cigarette consumption declined significantly in the United States. To help the cigarette industry, the U.S. government forced other countries, especially Asian countries, to open their borders to American cigarettes.

Some statistics suggest that more soldiers died from cigarette smoking after the war, and then soldiers actually died during the war. In 1994, heads of major tobacco companies testified before congress that evidence of cigarette smoking causing cancer and heart disease was inconclusive. Later, evidence from their own research indicated that they knew the health risks associated to smoking. Cigarette smokers are 2 to 4 times more likely to develop coronary heart disease than nonsmokers. Smoking doubles the risk of stroke (Source: Center of Disease Control).

So, it took 50 years to establish a causal relationship between smoking and heart disease. The tobacco industry was very resourceful. Smoking may well have been the main reason for the epidemic of heart disease after World War II, and not saturated fat and cholesterol.

CHAPTER 20

LIES, DAMNED LIES, STATISTICS (MARK TWAIN)

The holy grail of drug research is the double blind placebo controlled drug study. I participated in the physician health study that studied the effect of daily Aspirin use on the incidence of heart attacks.

The result: daily Aspirin use reduced the incidence of heart attacks by 40%. Now, it could be assumed that daily Aspirin use would also reduce mortality, but it does not. Why? We don't know, but the pharmaceutical industry suggested we should all take Aspirin to prevent heart attacks even it may increase death from other problems.

A large government sponsored study, the *Multiple Risk Factor Intervention Study* or *Mr. Fit* was a $115 million study started in 1973. Twelve thousand high-risk males with hypertension were split into two groups. The special intervention group was given antihypertensive medications (Diuretics) and was given intensive dietary counseling; the control group was given usual care, and they were told they were at high risk for heart disease. The study lasted 10 years. Sixty six percent of the special intervention group was able to normalize their blood pressure. After 10 years, an equal amount of patients died from both groups. The pharmaceutical industry spun the study in their favor, mainly: the medication lowered blood pressure successfully; therefore, patients with high blood pressure should take medications.

In 1987 the famous *Helsinki Heart Study* was published. A cholesterol lowering drug, gemfibrosil, was given to more than 4,000 patients. Cholesterol was lowered as much as 10%, and the number of heart attacks was lowered by 35%. Unfortunately, the treatment group and the control group had the same amount of deaths. This study was hailed as a triumph of medicine conquering heart disease. Little explanation was given for the fact that overall mortality did not change. An explanation for the lack of change in the mortality rate was never given by any of these studies. So why take a drug if the end result is the same?

These studies show that investigators can be biased, trying to promote their ideas and neglecting important parts of their study. And they know they have the full weight of the pharmaceutical industry behind them.

Conflict of interest is the trouble with drug studies, which are supposed to be unbiased. Many studies are observational studies that show correlation but not causation. According to the internet approximately 10,000 research studies are published every month. Nobody can keep up with this massive flow of information. The press picks up studies of interest. Which story sells? The press is not immune to bias. Oftentimes, what is sold as news is actually paid-advertising.

My pathology professor in medical school gave a lecture on observational studies. The incidence of lung cancer had steadily risen over the preceding 10 years. The number of television owners and car owners had risen the same way. This was statistically a clear correlation. But can owning a television or a car be the cause of lung cancer? This is quite unlikely. Many medical studies commit this

76

mistake of finding a correlation and thinking they have found the causal relationship.

For example, Dr. Burkitt a renowned physician, studied bowel habits in people in Africa. He found that tribes that consumed a lot of fiber and had multiple bowel movements every day had no colon cancer. This was a clear correlation. His assumption was that fibers prevent colon cancer (causation). He was influential; he wrote many papers and books and convinced a lot of people that a high fiber diet would prevent colon cancer. Now, forty years later and after many studies we know he was wrong. Yet the food industry continues to market some products under that theory.

The theory that a low fat diet prevents heart disease is based on correlation, and not causation. Ancel Keys studying dietary pattern of multiple populations in the world found a correlation in seven countries between saturated fat consumption, elevated cholesterol and heart disease. In 15 countries he could not demonstrate this correlation. Today, this study would probably never be accepted. In a way, this was scientific fraud. He was convincing and he wrote multiple papers with the government support. In fact, the government promised to fund multi-million dollar studies to prove his theory. The research departments of major universities were promised to be the recipients of this money. Keys' hypothesis was entirely unproven. But this was the beginning of the low fat heart healthy diet religion. No studies over the last 40 years have ever proven this theory. On the contrary, a low fat, high carbohydrate diet is thought by many to be the cause of the present epidemic of obesity and diabetes.

Many nutritional studies are not worth the paper they are written on. Two thousand journals are eager to accept papers and opinions. For example, after reviewing articles on coffee I found that some of the profound research findings were based on the experience with 6 or 8 patients. These kinds of publications cause confusion because what is the truth today will be contradicted with a different study in the future.

But even large studies from well-known universities are often only expressions of opinions. Let us look at the famous *Women's Health Initiative Study*. Twenty three thousand women were asked to follow a low fat, high fiber and high carbohydrate diet for eight years; they received psychological support and were advised to exercise regularly. A control group was told not to change their eating and exercise pattern. Cost of the study $1 billion.

The researchers were convinced that the experimental group of women would show major health benefits at the end of eight years; less cancer, less heart disease, less obesity and diabetes. The result was unexpected; the treated group had no health benefits compared to the control group. We could easily argue that the experimental protocol did not work. But we should never forget the human factor. Do we really know how many women followed the protocol? It is hard to believe that anybody can stick to an experimental protocol for eight years. They filled out multiple food questionnaires, they knew what the goal of the study was. Some did not stick to the diet but tried to please the researchers and answered the questions as expected from them. Those long term follow-up studies can never be truly scientific.

CHAPTER 21

FATS

There are three naturally occurring fats: monounsaturated fat, polyunsaturated fat and saturated fat. *Trans* fat is a fat artificially created by the food industry.

Trans Fat:

Trans fats are created when hydrogen is added to vegetable oil to make it more solid. Proctor and Gamble took advantage of this cheaper alternative to animal fat and created Crisco vegetable shortening. Crisco and similar fats were thought to be healthier than saturated fats. About 50 years ago saturated fats were thought to be the main culprit causing heart disease. *Trans* fats were promoted as a heart healthy alternative to saturated fat by our medical societies. Now it turns out they are far worse than butter or lard. *Trans* fats raise the bad cholesterol (LDL) and lower the good cholesterol (HDL). During a recent meeting on metabolism, Professor Rasmussen, a leading nutrition expert from Europe, was wondering how many people died due to this faulty recommendation *Trans* fats are found in fried and battered food, microwave popcorn, frozen desserts, frozen pizzas, cookies and pie crusts. According to the Grocery Manufactories Association, *trans* fats in food products have been reduced by 73% over the last 10 years .But this reduction is not enough. It is estimated by the FDA that eliminating all *trans* fats from our food supply could prevent 22,000 heart attacks per year. Just imagine how many heart attacks occurred before *trans* fats were reduced by 73%. The Diet of Hope is *trans* fat-free.

Saturated Fat:

Saturated fats were singled out as an important culprit in raising bad cholesterol (LDL), but later studies showed that they also raise good cholesterol (HDL). So, the ratio between good and bad cholesterol remains the same.

Also, there is a problem with the definition of saturated fat because most fats contain several different types. For example, 47% of lard is monounsaturated fat resembling olive oil, which is considered a healthy fat. Twelve percent is poly unsaturated fat like vegetable oil. Only 40% of lard is saturated fat and 30% of the 40% is stearic acid, acid that is found in chocolate and is considered a good fat. In sum, 70% of the fat in lard will improve our cholesterol profile and 30% raise the good and the bad cholesterol equally (Source: Gary Taubes). So why is lard called a saturated fat? Butter is 60% saturated 26% monounsaturated and 5% poly unsaturated and smaller amounts of other fats. Even olive oil contains 13% saturated fat. Coconut oil and palm oil have also been singled out as being damaging to the heart because they are saturated fats. They have a 12 carbon chain compared to the 18 carbon chain of most saturated fats. Populations who consume large amounts of these oils are healthy and with little heart disease.

Monounsaturated Fat:

Olives and olive oil, canola oil, peanut oil and most nuts, such as walnuts, almonds, cashews, and macadamia nuts are monounsaturated fats. Canola oil stands for Canadian oil low acid. Canola oil comes from rapeseed. Monounsaturated fats lower the bad cholesterol (LDL) and raise the good cholesterol (HDL).These fats are considered healthy. Olive oil is the most commonly used fat in Mediterranean countries. The island of Crete studied by Alan Keys in the Seven Country Study had the lowest rate of heart disease and the highest average life span. They had a higher consumption of fat than most other countries. Thirty seven percent of their calories came from fat mostly from olive oil, cheese, fish, meat and milk from grass fed animals and eggs from free range chickens.

The Lyon Heart Study compared the American low fat diet with the French diet that was higher in fat and also included some red wine. Six hundred patients with a heart attack were equally divided between the diets. The study was stopped when the patients on the low fat American diet had a 70% higher incidence of death from all causes.

Both studies suggest that consuming a low fat diet, which automatically is a high carbohydrate diet, is not healthy. Eating fats, especially the right fats, is important. The Diet of Hope promotes the consumption of good fats.

Polyunsaturated Fats:

The most important polyunsaturated fats are omega 3 and omega 6 fats. Those are fats that our body cannot produce; those are called essential fatty acids. Omega 6 and omega 3 should be in balance ideally in a one to one ratio, a more realistic ratio is three to one. Soybean oil has an omega 6 to omega 3 ratio of 10 to 1, corn oil a ratio of 100 to 1. We suggest avoiding corn, sunflower, cottonseed, grape seed, soybean and peanut oils. High omega 6 amount are also in meat from animals fed corn and soy, cows and pigs especially. Meat from grass fed animals has a good ratio of omega 6 to omega 3.

The American Heart Association has recently increased its dietary recommendation of omega 3 to three portions of fatty fish per week or 1 gram of omega 3 daily. Salmon, sardines, tuna, and herring are excellent sources of omega 3. In addition, there are now supplements available containing omega 3 extracted from grass and algae for vegetarians.

Before 1900, the production and dietary use of fats and oils derived from vegetable seeds was essentially zero. Not everybody believes they are healthy. Multiple steps are used in processing of seeds: cooking, mechanical pressing, solvent extraction, degumming, refining, bleaching, deodorizing. Fully processed oils are devoid of all nutrients present in the seeds. Processed oils are the equivalent of refined white sugar and can be called white oils. Like sugar, they are nutrient-deficient, provide mostly calories, but unlike sugar, may also contain toxins. For more information on this topic we recommend Udo Erasmus's book *Fats that Heal and Fats that Kill*.

The people on the island of Crete consumed more fat than Americans did in 1960, yet they had little heart disease. A major difference between Cretan and American diets lies in the consumption of sugar. In 1960 the average yearly consumption of sugar in Crete was 10 pounds, mostly from honey; the average consumption of sugar in the U.S. was 120 pounds.

CHAPTER 22

CHOLESTEROL

Cholesterol is a waxy substance essential for life. Cholesterol is a precursor of our sex hormones (testosterone and estrogen), and also a precursor of cortisone, and the hormones of the adrenal glands. Vitamin D is created from cholesterol. Twenty-five percent of myelin, an important insulator of the brain is cholesterol. So why is it thought to be the enemy?

Our thinking is based on numbers. A high cholesterol number is bad; we want it to be as low as possible. Some authorities try to make us believe that our cholesterol is high because of the absence of statins. The pharmaceutical industry has managed to convince some of our medical leaders of this notion. As a result, nobody is interested in other factors that cause our cholesterol to rise. Who cares, anyway? We have a pill for it!

Amazingly, some sanity has arrived at the American Heart Association and the College of Cardiology. They declared that no evidence exists that pushing our cholesterol number to the lowest level with drugs will improve our outcome. We apologize to the physician who tried hard to follow our advice, fearing a law suit if they didn't follow the gospel. The reality is that these misconceptions were simply opinions of leading scientist. We have now a new approach based on science. The new guidelines are:

- All patients with known heart disease should be on statins, nothing new.

- All diabetic patients should be on statins (nothing new).

We no longer push for certain cholesterol numbers. We look at the whole person, including their age, sex, race, blood pressure, and smoking history. We have a calculator which determines if patients should be on statins. Based on this calculator 30% of the adult population of the U.S. should be on statins. Not everybody agrees with this calculator. Certainly, I disagree. I am over 70 years old and white; the calculator tells me I should be on statins because of my age, even if I am otherwise perfectly healthy. What do they think my life expectancy is going to be? Maybe I can live a week longer on statins, but I will be exposed to all of the potential side effects of statins such as muscle pain, diabetes and brain fog.

We have a good Cholesterol (HDL) and a bad Cholesterol (LDL). I tell patients, H stands for healthy and L stands for lousy, which helps them remember. HDL should be above 40mg/dl in men and above 50mg/dl in women. Very high HDL levels were felt to be heart protective. Things are never straight forward. In Italy in a small village people live to a ripe old age with HDL's below 20mg/dl. Not all HDL is protective. Not all LDL is bad. LDL comes in a small dense form which is bad for our coronary arteries. The big fluffy form of LDL does little harm. Also, we can now count the number of particles of LDL and HDL. Our overall level of LDL might be acceptable, but if our number of small dense LDL particles is high we still might be in trouble.

Triglycerides are fat particles in our blood. A normal level of Triglycerides is considered to be below 150mg. High levels of

Triglycerides can also lead to heart disease and very high levels can cause inflammation of the pancreas.

Inflammatory markers are other significant risk factors known to damage our coronary arteries. The best known and most studied one is the high sensitive C-reactive protein (hs-crp). It should be below one. Our belly fat cells are known to produce multiple inflammatory substances. Fat cells not only store fat, their hormonal activities pose a significant health risk for our body.

Some scientists believe without inflammation of the inner lining of our arteries (called intima) cholesterol cannot damage our arteries. Statin drugs lower inflammation. This effect might actually be more important than lowering cholesterol. A low fat-diet predictably lowers HDL, raises triglycerides and changes LDL to the small dense form.

Our Diet of Hope helps raise HDL, lowers triglycerides sometimes dramatically, changes LDL to the more fluffy form and helps lower inflammation.

CHAPTER 23

THE EGG STORY

The great crusade against cholesterol-rich food started 40 years ago. Eggs became public enemy number one because one egg contains 200mg of cholesterol. Three ounces of beef, pork or chicken contain only 70mg to 80mg of cholesterol. Now the food authorities are allowing us to eat eggs again, but with limits. It is recommended our daily consumption of cholesterol should not exceed 300mg if we are healthy. So, one egg a day or less should be the limit. After researching the literature I did not find a single study demonstrating that eating eggs causes heart disease. The Harvard Egg Study showed no ill effects amongst a group of volunteers eating one egg daily. In fact, this group's cholesterol numbers did not change.

A government survey showed that men over 65 cut egg consumption by 46% because of the cholesterol scare. Eggs can provide the elderly with an inexpensive nutritious food. In a study from the University of Connecticut, 42 patients 60 years or older were given 3 eggs daily for one month. Both the good and the bad cholesterol rose minimally. The particle size of the bad Cholesterol (LDL) increased and it became fluffier, which is healthy.

Then there is the 1991 study in the New England Journal. A Colorado man age 88 was observed to have eaten 25 eggs per day for at least 5 years (possibly 15 years). He had normal cholesterol levels, and did not have heart disease. His liver had markedly reduced cholesterol production. In addition, he absorbed only 18% of the cholesterol he consumed, he doubled the conversion of cholesterol to bile acid part of it was excreted in his stool. A study done at the same time with 11 volunteers eating 5 eggs per day showed that they only absorbed 50% of the cholesterol eaten.

Most nutritionists that believe in independent thinking support the concept that eating cholesterol containing food does not cause an elevation of blood cholesterol, nor does it cause heart disease.

Elevated insulin levels related to a high refined-carbohydrate diet stimulate the liver to produce cholesterol. Insulin stimulates an enzyme called HMG CoA reductase (3-hydroxy-3-methyl-glutaryl-CoA reductase). This is the same enzyme that statin drugs block from producing cholesterol.

The Nutritional Value of Eggs
(Based on one large egg)
- 75 calories
- Protein 6.5gm
- Fat 5gm
- Carbohydrates 0

Protein

The egg's protein contains all the essential amino acids, and is easy to digest.

Fat

47% of an egg's fat is monounsaturated (like olive oil), 23% is polyunsaturated (omega3 and omega6), eggs from free range chicken have a higher omega 3 level, and 32% of the fat is saturated.

Vitamins

Eggs contain all vitamins except vitamin C. Eggs are an especially good source for vitamin B12, B2 and folate. Egg yolk is a rare source of vitamin D; it is also rich in Vitamin A.

Lutein and Zeaxanthin in part responsible for the yellow color of the egg yolk are important for our eye health. They may be helpful in the treatment of age related macular degeneration (AMD).

Lecithin

Eggs are one of the richest sources of Lecithin a phospholipid present in every body cell. Some studies have suggested that it can block cholesterol absorption in the gut.

Minerals

Eggs are a rich source of iodine (for thyroid), iron, selenium, zinc (important for wound healing) and phosphorus (bone health). In addition, eggs are rich source of choline. Choline consumption has shown to improve cardiovascular health.

The Perfect Food

Eggs are a perfect food. Cholesterol in eggs was condemned before we understood how the body deals with it. From my own research, I have concluded that cholesterol in eggs cause no health problems. Most breakfasts in our Diet of Hope start with eggs. Eggs provide satiety and good nutrition. Breakfast cereals provide neither.

CHAPTER 24

PROTEIN

The three macronutrients in our food are protein, fat, and carbohydrates. Proteins are the most important nutrients. The building blocks for proteins are amino acids. There are 20 amino acids; 9 amino acids are called essential because our body cannot create them, they must come from food.

Our human body is made mostly of protein: muscles, hair, skin, blood, nerves, bones, and organs. There is a continuous breakdown and repair of proteins. For this reason we need a steady supply of high quality protein. We have animal proteins and vegetable proteins. Animal proteins are the most complete proteins, meaning they have all the nine essential amino acids, while vegetable proteins are often incomplete proteins. Several different vegetables need to be combined to obtain a full complement of essential amino acids.

With the Diet of Hope we emphasize the importance of protein for a healthy diet. Proteins preserve the lean body mass. Also, proteins reduce heart disease and provide satiety. As a snack or a meal replacement, we utilize protein drinks. The protein in these drinks is whey protein, which is a by-product of cheese production. Whey consumption has several benefits: it raises the good cholesterol HDL, it does not contain lactose, and it is easily digested. Whey is a complete protein.

All proteins have a thermo genic effect; they increase the basic metabolic rate which contributes to weight control. Approximately 10%of the calories of protein are used in the process of their metabolism.

The minimum daily need for protein has been calculated at approximately 0.5gm per pound of body weight or 100gm for a person weighing 200 pounds. Four ounces of meat or chicken contain 25gm of protein; four ounces of fish contain 18gm of protein and one egg 7gm to 8gm. The maximum amount of protein the body can digest is not clear. Doubling the minimum amount of protein to 1gm per pound of body weight appears to be safe. For people with a very high percentage of body fat this may be too much.

The Inuit of the Arctic (Eskimos) were intensely studied 60 years ago. They were healthy, with very little evidence of heart disease, diabetes, cancer and kidney problems. Their diet consists of 30%protein and 70% fat. On average, they consume 3,000 calories per day 900 calories or 225gm will come from protein.

Our program provides sufficient, but not excessive protein. There is still a fear that higher protein consumption causes kidney problems. To my knowledge, no evidence exists that a high protein intake damages a healthy kidney. Actually, we have observed that some patients with mild renal dysfunction improved their kidney function on our diet.

Some of the criticisms of a diet higher in protein are based on studies that the urine becomes more acidic and calcium is excreted through the urine to neutralize the acidity. Newer studies suggest that with a higher protein intake more calcium will be absorbed. We emphasize to our patients to increase the intake of non-starchy vegetables. Vegetables are mostly alkaline. This would balance the pH in blood and urine (refer to the chapter on pH).

The new food plate from the United States Department of Agriculture (USDA) suggests we should get approximately 25% of our calories from protein. A patient eating 3,000 calories per day, which is common in our patients, can eat 750 calories from protein or 187gm.

We calculate the amount of protein need for our patients based on sex, height, weight and age. Given that we significantly restrict simple carbohydrates, the percentage of protein per meal is higher, but the total amount is in the acceptable range.

CHAPTER 25

MASAI AND ESKIMOS

The Masai and Eskimos are two cultures on high fat diets, and both groups are healthy, free of heart disease and cancer.

In 1964, a field study among 400 Masai men, women and children revealed they had no clinical heart disease, had low cholesterol levels and low blood pressure (Source: Journal of Atherosclerosis Research 4: 289-312.)

In 2000, my wife and I were invited to spent time with a Masai tribe in Tanzania. We had the opportunity to observe their daily life activities and their eating habits. Their diet consists primarily of milk, blood and meat. Masais are tall and slim, both men and women. We were invited to a 3 day hiking trip to visit a neighboring tribe. Our food supply consisted of two goats walking with us. The Masais had a cup of milk for breakfast and ate nothing during the day. In the evening a goat was slaughtered. The Masais first drank the blood from the goat, than each tribal member consumed a piece of raw liver and kidneys. Afterwards, they joined us in eating the roasted meat. The meal ended with a soup made from the bark of an Acacia tree. Masais are slim and strong; hiking 20 to 30 miles a day is no problem for them. On the contrary, we had problems keeping up with them. We thought we were in top shape since we had recently climbed Kilimanjaro.

Interestingly, Masais do not hunt. They only eat meat from cows, sheep and goats. Only recently have they been introduced to agriculture. Their living space has become more and more restricted. Their nomadic live is coming to an end.

Couples are only allowed to marry after the big rains when their cows can eat the best grass and their milk is the healthiest. This would guarantee the health of the couple's baby.

The only person in the village with a belly was the village chief. When we asked what we could do for him and the village, his answer was to send him Coca Cola.

Eskimos are another example of people who eat a very high fat diet without showing signs of heart disease and cancer. The Eskimos in the Arctic were intensely studied by an anthropologist from Canada, Vilhjalmur Stefansson, who spent 5 years living with the Eskimos. On average, the food of an Eskimo consists of 70% fat and 30% protein (50% Caribou, 30% fish, 10% seal meat, and 5% to 10% polar bears, birds and eggs). They have no access to carbohydrates, vegetables and fruits. They showed no evidence of vitamin deficiencies, especially scurvy. Speculations as to where Eskimos get their vitamins range from raw adrenal glands of the caribou to fatty meats to willow bark. Eskimos had no evidence of diabetes, heart disease, high blood pressure or cancer. What is more, their cholesterol levels were normal.

In the December edition of Harper's Magazine (1935), Stevansson described a yearlong stay at the Bellevue Hospital in New York eating an Eskimo diet under close supervision. He had no ill effects, he felt strong and his cholesterol changed little. The only time he became ill was when the researchers changed his diet from fatty meat to lean meat. He developed diarrhea and lost significant weight. This problem was quickly corrected when he was allowed again to eat fatty meat.

In recent times, Eskimos have become exposed to a western diet and developed all the diseases of western civilization, such as diabetes, cancer and heart disease.

CHAPTER 26

PH AND BONE HEALTH

PH is a measure of acidity or alkalinity of a solution. The pH of blood and body fluids is 7.4, a pH below 7.35 is called acidosis, and a pH above 7.45 is called alkalosis. Our body functions best with a pH of 7.4. Acidosis depresses our nervous systems and extreme acidosis can lead to death. Alkalosis causes hyper excitability of our nervous system and muscles that can lead to seizures and death.

Why is the pH of food important? If acidic food dominates in our diet our body needs to neutralize the acid with alkaline substances from our body. Calcium carbonate and specifically calcium phosphate from our bones are used to balance the blood pH. Excessive consumption of acidic food over a long period of time can lead to osteoporosis.

In a healthy body the blood pH remains stable at 7.4. Our food can influence the pH of our blood. For example, carbonated sodas are dietary sources of acid; Coca-Cola contains phosphoric acid. Most carbonated sodas have a pH of 3.

Protein from all animal products are acidic; milk and cheeses are acidic, especially parmesan cheese. The digestion of animal proteins yields sulfuric acid and uric acid.

Wheat and oats are among the most potent sources of sulfuric acid (William Davis MD). Grains such as wheat account for 38% of acid load in a typical American diet. Most food in the produce department such as spinach, cabbage, kale and most fruits are alkaline.

Our Diet of Hope creates a neutral pH by combining acidic animal products with alkaline vegetables and avoiding highly acidic grains and sodas.

Milk is an acidic food. Regular milk has a pH of 6.7; skim milk has a pH of 5.1 to 5.7.   Consuming milk that contains a significant amount of calcium may not be the answer for osteoporosis (see chapter on milk).

An adequate consumption of protein is important for bone health. Protein also stimulates the production of a substance in our body called IGF1 (Insulin like growth factor), important for bone growth.

CHAPTER 27

GOT MILK?

Milk is advertised with slick commercials .When most people in the United States think about milk, they instantly think about calcium. Milk calcium is supposedly good for our bones, according to the milk industry. One cup of milk provides 300mg of calcium, one cup of cooked spinach 240mg, one cup cooked broccoli 180mg. How much does the body need? The US government recommends 1,000 to 1,200mg per day. In England, the recommended dose is 700mg. In India, Japan, Peru the daily consumption of calcium is close to 300mg. Those countries have a very low incidence of osteoporosis and bone fractures. In order to get the recommended amount of calcium in the US we would have to drink 3 cups of milk which would add 438 extra calories to our diet. Instead, why don't we simply take a Vitamin D supplement? A Vitamin D supplement has no calories and it helps the bones. Whether milk helps the bones still remains an unsettled question.

How Healthy is Milk?

Milk is designed as food source for neonates. Grown-ups frequently are intolerant to Lactose, the milk sugar. Ninety percent of Asians are unable to digest Lactose, 75% of Native Americans and African Americans are intolerant to Lactose, while Northern Europeans have a better tolerance.

Lactose consists of two sugars, Galactose and Glucose. To split the sugars we need an enzyme Lactase, if the sugar is not split in the small intestine it reaches the colon and produces diarrhea, bloating and gas.

Milk has 4% protein, 3.3% fat and 4% lactose. One cup of whole milk has 146 calories; 39% come from fat, 30% from carbohydrates and 21% from protein.

On average, a calf weighs 80 pounds at birth. It gains two pounds a day or doubles its weight in 40 days consuming his mother's milk (fresh unpasteurized milk). So if we want to grow like calves, then we should drink a lot of milk.

A patient of mine, who is a cattle farmer, shared an interesting fact about milk. In the case of a mother cow dying, and her calf is fed pasteurized milk, the calf will die. However, if one raw egg is added to the orphan calf's milk every day, the calf will live. According to our government, pasteurization does not affect the nutritional quality of milk. Why would the calf die if the milk is not changed by pasteurization?

What is pasteurization? Milk is being heated to 160 degrees Fahrenheit for 30 seconds and then quickly cooled. Pasteurization is done to kill harmful bacteria, but it also destroys some important proteins. This process prolongs the shelf life of the milk substantially, a major benefit for the milk industry.

In 1993, the FDA approved Monsanto to use recombinant bovine growth hormone (rBGH) in order to stimulate more milk production. More milk requires more milking, which causes more udder infections (mastitis). To treat the infections antibiotics are used. Both growth hormone and antibiotics can end up in milk.

The European Union has banned growth hormones because of the lack of information regarding the potential side effects of consuming milk that may contain growth hormone for a long period of time.

Studies from Harvard University (Nurses' Health Study) showed a 44% higher risk for ovarian cancer in women consuming milk frequently compared to infrequent milk drinkers. Results from the Physician Health Study found that high intake of dairy products and calcium increased the risk of prostate cancer. The latest study from Harvard University found a high level of estrone sulfate (a hormone-like substance) in pasteurized milk from industrially produced milk, a possible link to testicular, prostate and breast cancer (Source: Dr. Ganmaa Davaasambuu). Milk from grass fed cows had low levels of estrone sulfate.

CHAPTER 28

BREAKFAST CEREALS: FOOD FOR THE TOOTHLESS

John Harvey Kellogg is considered to be the inventor of breakfast cereals. He was a physician in charge of a sanatorium in Michigan, owned by Seventh Day Adventists. He promoted a vegetarian diet. Kellogg was experimenting with grains to create an easily digestible food that sick and toothless people could eat. In addition, he thought grains would reduce the urge to masturbate, as he was a most ardent anti-masturbator.

He cooked wheat and afterwards rolled it out in thin layers. One day, the cooked wheat was left unattended, and hours later it had significantly softened. When the wheat was rolled, each little wheat grain separated like a flake. The flakes turned out to be tasty cereals. Dr. Kellogg patented the process in 1894.

His brother W.K. Kellogg recognized the commercial potential. His major contribution to the creation of cereals was adding sugar, which most people preferred to the unsweetened cereals. Dr. Kellogg was vehemently opposed to the addition of sugar. The brothers separated, each started a separate company. Obviously, the sugar cereals were a big hit and gained popularity. The brothers became enemies and each went their own way.

W.K. Kellogg started a massive advertising campaign, and ever since then cereals with added sugar have become the breakfast choice.

General Mills created Cheerios and started to advertise their cereals as heart healthy. In one obscure study financed by General Mills, but considered an independent study, cholesterol levels lowered by four percent after six weeks. I could not find the original study. I would have liked to know what else the study participants ate and did.

Some studies exist that have shown lowering cholesterol reduces heart disease. General Mills felt justified to advertise "our cereals reduce heart disease". The FDA intervened in 2009 and told General Mills that such claims required scientific support. Now, General Mills advertises that cereals could be part of a heart healthy diet and could reduce the risk of heart disease.

Most cereals are made from refined grains and end up in our blood stream as sugar very quickly. Cereals made from whole grain have a bit more nutrition, but their blood sugar response is not much different from refined cereals. There are multiple different Cheerios cereals, most have regular sugar added. In my opinion, cereals should not be used by diabetics or obese people.

The Diet of Hope recommends eggs for breakfast. Patients on our program for 6 weeks lower their cholesterol on average 12%.

CHAPTER 29

WHEAT

Wheat Belly, written by Dr. William Davis, became a number one New York Times bestseller. It is a worthwhile read, and our Diet of Hope fully supports its conclusions. Our program is wheat and gluten free.

The dietary recommendations from the United States Department of Agriculture (USDA) have become a bit more sophisticated since the publication of the food pyramid in 1992. However, the food plate is still strongly recommending the consumption of whole wheat bread, cereals, pasta, muffins and other whole wheat products. According to the USDA, we are supposed to eat at least three servings of whole wheat daily. Refined wheat is no longer in. What is the difference between refined and whole? A kernel of grain has three layers, an outer layer that is fiber and has some vitamins and minerals (bran), a middle layer that is mostly sugar (endosperm) and an inner core (germ), which hast most of the nutrition including good fats. The fats become rancid during storage. Refining means eliminating the inner nutritious core, and also destroying the outer fiber layer in the process. This refined flour can be stored for a long time without spoiling. Because the flour is devoid of nutrition, our government forced the bread and cereal makers to add some vitamins to the end product.

To increase shelf life of whole wheat bread, preservatives such as calcium propionate, sodium propionate or sulfur dioxide are used. Additionally, most bread has sugar and salt added.

The modern wheat flour is 70% carbohydrate by weight, 15% protein and 15% fiber. Of the complex carbohydrates in wheat 75% is amylopectin and 25%amylose. Amylopectin consists of branching glucose molecules. Amylopectin is speedily digested by an enzyme amylase to glucose. This efficient digestion is the reason why whole wheat has a high glycemic index of 72. Regular table sugar (sucrose) has a glycemic index of 59. We consider wheat a complex carbohydrate, but because it is so quickly digested it acts like a simple carbohydrate.

Eating whole wheat causes a fast and steep rise of blood sugar, similar to drinking a can of sugary soda. This fast rise in blood sugar triggers a significant insulin response. Insulin is a storage hormone, and some of that sugar ends up as belly fat. Whole wheat for some people is addictive, acting almost like a drug. Wheat is a potent source of sulfuric acid. Grains contribute a significant acid load to the average American diet.

Our body does well without eating "Healthy Whole Grain". It is a total myth that our body needs grains. The Diet of Hope provides a healthy alternative: plenty of none starchy vegetables, all types of meat (preferable grass fed), fish and fowl, eggs, good fats, nuts, olives, and cheese.

CHAPTER 30

GLUTEN

Gluten has been joining cholesterol and *trans* fat as something undesirable in our food. The food industry obliged quickly with offering gluten free food made out of cornstarch, rice starch, potato starch or tapioca. This food is basically refined sugar of little nutritional value. On the other hand, our medical societies and dietitians promote whole wheat, which contains gluten as health food. Gluten occurs in wheat, rye, barley, spelt, bulgur and kamut. Wheat is the main carbohydrate most people consume. For breakfast we eat pancakes, waffles, French toast, cereals, muffins, bagels and toast.

What is gluten? Gluten is a protein that makes wheat doughy, stretchable and twistable. It allows the dough to rise when yeast fermentation causes it to fill with air pockets. Rice flour or corn flour doesn't have this property. Glutens are the storage protein for the wheat plant. Gluten consists of two protein families, the gliadins and the glutenins. The gliadins are mostly responsible for the immune reaction that causes celiac disease. The glutens provoke an immune response in the small intestines causing severe inflammation that produces severe abdominal cramping and diarrhea. It is estimated that 1 in 130 persons have celiac disease.

It is believed that many more people are sensitive to gluten, but do not show the severe changes in the intestines.

The trouble is that a definite diagnosis is difficult to establish. Symptoms thought to be related to gluten are multiple, ranging from irritable bowel syndrome to fibromyalgia, joint pains, arthritis, asthma, acid reflux and diffuse neurological symptoms (brain fog). At times eliminating gluten for a month may help with the diagnoses.

Celiac disease can be suggested by three different antibody tests.

1. Antigliadin antibodies: they fail to diagnose 20 to 50% of true celiac disease.
2. Transglutaminase antibody: this antibody can identify approximately 85%of celiac cases.
3. Endomysium antibody: this antibody identifies close to 90% of celiac cases.

Small intestinal biopsy is the gold standard for the diagnoses of celiac disease. Genetic markers for human leukocyte antigen HLADQ2 and HLADQ8 are found in over 90% of celiac disease sufferers. The Diet of Hope is gluten free.

CHAPTER 31

FREQUENTLY ASKED QUESTIONS

Alcohol

Alcoholism is defined as a pattern of drinking that results in harm to one's health, interferes with personal relationships and ability to work. For the majority of people, alcohol consumption in moderation is beneficial. US Government Dietary Guidelines support moderate drinking. The definition of moderate drinking is two drinks a day for men and one drink for women. Clearly, this is a case of gender discrimination! Body size is probably more important in alcohol tolerance. A 12 ounce beer, a 5 ounce glass of wine, a 1.5 ounce of hard liquor contain 0.6 ounce of alcohol. The calorie content in each is different. A 12 ounce beer has 150 calories, a light beer 110 calories, a glass of wine 90 to 100 calories, and a Piña Colada (9 ounces) has 480 calories.

First, let's discuss the bad problems associated with excessive alcohol consumption:

Alcohol increases the risk of liver cirrhosis, cancer of the esophagus and other gastrointestinal cancers, raises blood pressure and the risk of stroke. Heavy drinking for a long period of time causes shrinking of the brain, resulting in dementia.

The Good News:

Moderate drinking of any kind of alcohol reduces the risk of heart disease (US Government Dietary Guidelines). It raises our good cholesterol (HDL). Moderate drinking in early adult life may reduce the risk of dementia later in life.

Older and middle-aged moderate drinkers will outlive nondrinkers by reducing death from all causes (Source: November 2010 issue of Alcoholism: Clinical and Experimental Research).

Of all the alcoholic drinks, red wine consumption produces the most benefits. Red wine is loaded with antioxidants, flavonoids and especially resveratrol. Moderate consumption of red wine is good for the heart (Source: American Heart Association). A glass of red wine daily reduces the risk of aggressive prostate cancer by half (National Cancer Institute).

The French on average have a higher cholesterol level than Americans do, however they have only half the incident of heart attacks (The French paradox). One of the theories states it is the regular consumption of red wine that makes the difference. Who knows? During our phase one of our Diet of Hope we suggest not to drink alcohol, since alcohol has calories. We want our patients to be very successful in those first 6 weeks because success is a great confidence builder.

Coffee

Some are trying hard to show the beneficial effects of coffee, while others see it as the devil's beverage. Below are several beneficial effects of coffee that have been published (Source: Internet):

- Increased intelligence

- Improves physical performance (Athletes)

- Reduces the risk of type 2 diabetes

- Coffee reduces the risk of dying

- Coffee is loaded with nutrients and antioxidants

- Coffee helps burn fat

- Coffee may reduce the risk of Alzheimer's disease and Parkinson's disease

Negative Effects of Coffee:

- Acid reflux and heart burn can be caused by coffee. Coffee stimulates stomach acid production.

- Coffee can cause diarrhea

- Acrylamide is formed when coffee beans are roasted at high temperature. Acryl amide is potentially carcinogenic

- Caffeine can be addictive

We have to realize scientific studies are not always scientific. Epidemiological studies can show correlation, but not cause. Most coffee studies are epidemiological studies.

My Recommendation:

Enjoy a cup or two in the morning; forget the sugar, forget the milk and use whole cream. Tea is also a good alternative to coffee.

Chocolate: The Delicious News

The health benefits of chocolate, especially dark chocolate, have recently been discovered. Chocolate contains flavenols (antioxidants) that reduce cell damage implicated in heart disease. Flavenols reduce blood pressure and improve vascular function. Some studies have suggested that chocolate consumption reduces the risk of diabetes, stroke and heart attack. This data reflect studies with dark chocolate, the cocoa content should be 65% or higher.

My Recommendation:

Chocolate studies are in fashion right now. All the beneficial results are based on short term studies. The fat content in an ounce of chocolate is 150 calories, and for this reason chocolate should be used sparingly.

Artificial Sweeteners:

All the health gurus on the internet are strongly against artificial sweeteners. However, they have not shown us any real data. So, it is their personal opinion. The FDA has cleared Splenda and Stevia, our preferred sweeteners. The sugar industry keeps a close eye on the competition. If there would be a real proven problem with these sweeteners it is guaranteed that we would know about any issues immediately.

Most people who drink diet sodas rarely lose weight. My theory is that anything sweet entering our mouth alerts the brain of possible sugar coming in. The brain in turn signals the pancreas to release some insulin, which is fine if real sugar comes in. But, if the sweetener is not sugar, then there might be a small drop in blood sugar. This drop may cause hunger.

Can We Overdose on Water?

We are told that we should all drink at least 8 tall glasses of water every day. Everyone, young or old, carries a water bottle if they go for a little walk, go to the movies, go to the opera, just in case. The message that the body needs 8 tall glasses of water appears to be universally accepted.

However, drinking too much water can also be harmful, marathon runners have died because of water intoxication. Several of our patients ended up in the emergency room because of very low sodium and potassium level related to over-consumption of water. We need to understand that the need for water is different for each of us. If we live in an air conditioned environment we need much less water than somebody who works in the outdoors.

I tried to find the original source of this "8 glasses per day" recommendation and found research performed by the Swiss Army. Young soldiers were studied on Monte Rosa Mountain in Switzerland training at an altitude of 14,000 feet. In order for the soldiers to stay in water balance they were required to drink 8 tall glasses of water daily.

My Recommendation:

We should listen to our body, drink water when thirsty and check our urine color (clear urine is fine). Like always, too much of a good thing can be a bad thing.

Vitamin D the Sunshine Vitamin:

Depending what source you use 30 to 50% of all adults are vitamin D deficient. In our practice, at least 80% of patients are Vitamin D deficient. A normal vitamin D level should be above 30ng/dl (some people argue it should be above 45ng/dl). Vitamin D is the most studied vitamin ever. Last year my wife attended a seminar just on vitamin D. One thing we know is that it cures rickets. A teaspoon of castor oil (made from salmon liver) contains 400 units of vitamin D.

Official daily vitamin recommendations are 600 IU for people under 70 and 800 IU for people above 70. Many researchers suggest using a significantly higher dose. Low levels of vitamin D have been associated with a multitude of diseases: Multiple Scleroses, Rheumatoid Arthritis, Heart Disease and most Modern Nutritional Diseases.

Researchers from the University in Salt Lake City followed 27,868 people age 50 and older for more than one year and found that people with a very low vitamin D level were 77% more likely to die compared to people with a high normal vitamin D level. A large cohort study published in the American Journal of Clinical Nutrition (2013 97:782-793) showed a strong correlation between low vitamin D levels and all causes of mortality, including cardiovascular disease, cancer and respiratory disease.

Where does vitamin D come from? It is very difficult to obtain adequate vitamin D from food sources, most animal food sources have very small amounts and plants have none, except for some mushrooms.

The main source for Vitamin D is sunshine. UV lights triggers the production of a precursor of vitamin D in our skin from cholesterol. Our liver and kidneys than create the full vitamin.

The dermatologists have convinced everybody that sun will kill them, especially in Arizona. Nobody goes outdoors without a big layer of protective sunscreen. Only the tourists have color, native Arizonans are pale.

My Recommendation:

I suggest try to get daily sun exposure for at least 15 minutes or longer (without sunscreen), after a while tolerance builds up. I am not sure why almost all of our overweight patients have a low level of vitamin D. My assumption is that since vitamin D dissolves in fat, maybe fat cells have become a storage place for vitamin D.

FEATURED RECIPES

We are including a few recipes from the Diet of Hope program and from patients, employees and family

"HEALTH STARTS WITH THE FOOD YOU EAT"

Raquel's Famous Chile Rellenos

Raquel puts a special twist to Chile Rellenos. After tasting this version of Chile Rellenos you will never go back to regular ones. These are great for entertaining and can be made ahead.

Ingredients

6 Roasted and cleaned green chiles
One 16oz can whole tomatoes
4 eggs separate white from yolk
8oz Cheddar and Jack Shredded cheese
2 fresh tomatoes
½ Cup chopped white onion
½ cup fresh chopped cilantro
 ½ teaspoon minced garlic
½ cup olive oil
Salt and Pepper to taste

Directions

1. Wisk the egg white until frothy **2**. Slowly introduced the egg yolk to the egg white **3**. Slit each Chile open remove seeds and stuff with ½ to ¾ cup shredded cheese **4**. Heat up oil in a frying pan
5. Take each Chile and dip into egg mixture making sure to cover them completely **6**. Place each Chile in the frying pan with ½ of the olive oil and roast each one until egg is cooked **6**. Remove from pan and place in a deep serving platter **7**. Place canned tomatoes and garlic and blend (don't over blend) **8**. Using the same frying pan add the remainder olive oil and sauté the onions **9**. Slowly add the blended tomatoes and continue to cook until piping hot **10**. When ready to remove from the fire, add fresh chopped tomatoes and cilantro **11**. Pour mixture over the Chile rellenos and serve.
Servings will vary calculate between 2-3 Chiles per person

Submitted by Raquel Gonzalez

Toni's Stuffed Portabella Mushrooms

These are delicious and great for entertaining.

Ingredients

2 Fresh portabella mushrooms
2 Tablespoon Olive Oil
3 Cloves minced garlic
2 Green Onion, sliced thinly
8 ounces ground turkey
½ cup low sodium beef stock
Salt and Pepper to taste

Directions

1. Heat a skillet on medium heat, add olive oil, garlic and green onions until they are sauté and softened **2.** Add ground turkey, salt and pepper to taste and cook until it's brown, Stir occasionally **3.** Set aside to cool.

4. Preheat oven to 350 degrees. **5.** Remove any stems from mushrooms **6.** Fill cap of portabella mushroom and place in a baking dish. Add ½ cup beef stock inside the dish. Cover with foil and place in oven. Cook for 30 minutes. Serves 2.

Submitted by Toni Cruz

Turkey Sloppy Gobblers

"I just eat my dad's cooking and lost almost 100 lbs"

Quote by Shannon Pfleiderer

Ingredients:

1 medium Onion, Raw (diced)
1 medium Green Bell Pepper (diced)
2 cloves Garlic (finely diced)
1 Tbsp Italian Seasoning
3/4 pound Lean Ground Turkey
1-1/2 tsp A1 Steak Sauce
1-1/2 tsp Lite Soy Sauce
1 cup Traditional Spaghetti Sauce (Prego)

Directions

1. In a hot dry skillet over medium heat, dry sauté the onion, bell pepper and garlic until slightly browned, 3-5 minute. Stir in the Italian Seasoning.
2. To the skillet add the ground turkey, stirring to break up and cooked through and browned.
3. Reduce the heat to medium-low stir in steak sauce, soy sauce, Cover pan (open the vent) and simmer 8-10 minutes. Do not let the mixture boil.
Servings: 6

Submitted by GPFleiderer

Glenna's Choice Gazpacho

Glenna calls this choice because the ingredients and quantity are your choice. She makes enough at each batch to last two weeks. Not only does she eat it as a cold soup, but also uses it as a base for dishes with protein.

Ingredients

Diced canned tomatoes (1 gallon)
4 large bell peppers red, orange and yellow for color and vitamins
3 English cucumbers

Optional Ingredients

Sweet Banana Peppers (I don't like spicy foods so I use these)
Hot Peppers (My husband prefers spicy so I add these)
Pepper juice from peppers (to taste)
Onions
Salt, pepper, garlic to taste

Directions

1. Place canned tomatoes in an empty container with lid that can remain in our refrigerator **2**. Chop the bell peppers into quarter to half inch size **3**. Peel the cucumbers and cut into four quarters then slice **4**. Cut the peppers and onion into small pieces **5**. Add to the container **6**. Add the juice from the peppers **7**. Add salt, pepper to taste. **8**. Stir and refrigerate.

The Gazpacho will taste best if it has 24 hours to marinate in the refrigerator before it is served

Submitted by Glenna Kornegay

Cheryl's Flourless Chocolate Cake

Great way to celebrate birthdays or special occasions guilt

Ingredients

1 cup butter
8 ounces Semisweet chocolate chips
¾ cup Stevia or Splenda
1 cup Sifted unsweetened cocoa powder
6 large eggs
10" spring form pan
Parchment paper

Directions

1. Butter the spring form pan **2**. Line bottom with parchment paper **3**. Stir butter and chocolate chips in heavy saucepan on low heat until melted **4**. Mix stevia and cocoa in large bowl
5. Add eggs, whisk until blended **6**. Whisk in chocolate/butter mixture **7**. Pour batter into prepared pan **8**. Bake at 350 degrees for 45 minutes

Cool cake completely in pan on rack
Turn knife around pan sides to loosen
Release pan sides - cover and refrigerate

Submitted by Cheryl Parker

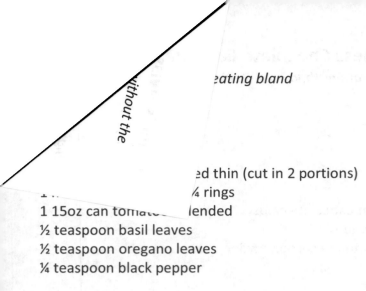

eating bland

ed thin (cut in 2 portions)
¼ rings
1 15oz can tomatoes blended
½ teaspoon basil leaves
½ teaspoon oregano leaves
¼ teaspoon black pepper

Directions

1. Brown steak in pam sprayed non-stick pan on both sides **2.** Top with onion circles **3**. Pour blended tomatoes on top and add seasonings **4**. Cover and simmer for 30 to 40 minutes.
You may serve over baked spaghetti squash.

Submitted by Elaine Silverness

Diet of Hope Chipotle Garlic Shrimp

If you enjoy spicy food this is a great dish

Ingredients

1 pound medium shrimp deveined shelled
4-6 cloves of garlic peeled and crushed
1 small can (7oz) chipotle chile
1/8 cup lime juice
Salt and pepper to taste
Chopped cilantro for garnish

Directions

1. Deseed chipotle chile and place in blender until finely minced
2. Add lime juice and garlic blend all ingredients together
3. In a large plastic bag or Tupperware place shrimp and pour in minced chipotle sauce **4**. Shake until all shrimp are covered with the chipotle sauce.
You may grill, fry or bake this dish (be careful not to overcook shrimp)
If you wish to bake heat oven to 325 degrees and bake for 15 minutes or until shrimp is done

Diet of Hope Mushroom Goulash Delight

(Meatless version substitute 1 lb. of mushrooms in place of meat)

Ingredients

8oz cubed meat (beef, pork, lamb)
2 large bell peppers seeded and cubed (use different color)
½ lb. wild or button mushrooms
1 cup chopped leeks.
1/2 medium coarsely chopped onion
1-2 garlic cloves minced.
4-6 Tablespoons hot Hungarian paprika
One 16 oz can of diced tomatoes.
4 cups low sodium vegetable broth
3 Tablespoons extra virgin olive oil.
Salt and pepper to taste

Directions

1. In a large skillet heat 2 tablespoons of olive oil and brown the meat **2.** In separate soup pot start heating the 4 cups of broth **3**. When meat is browned remove from skillet and place in soup pot. **4.** Place onion, garlic, leeks, bell peppers in same skillet you browned meat in and sauté until onions are translucent
5. Remove all ingredients from skillet and carefully place in soup pot.
6. Add the remaining 1 tablespoon of oil and sauté the mushrooms until golden **7**. Add mushrooms to the soup pot
8. Add the paprika (if you desire use more or less paprika) to the diced tomatoes and stir into the soup pot **9**. Cook for about 45 minutes on low heat.
Hint: instead of salt I always use low sodium bouillon paste for flavor
        If desired after you have browned and sautéed ingredients you can place them in a crock pot to cook.

Spinach Lasagna Diet of Hope Style

Don't tell anyone this is healthy for them, they will never know the difference! Enjoy!

Ingredients

2 lbs Ground Meat
2 16oz cans Tomato paste (to taste)
1 onion chopped
1 16oz can stewed tomatoes (drained)
½-1 lb mushrooms chopped
16 oz shredded mozzarella cheese
1 lb Ricotta Cheese
2 lb fresh uncooked spinach
Italian spices, pepper and salt to taste
Fresh garlic

Directions

1. In large pot sauté onions and mushrooms until onions are translucent **2**. Remove from heat and place in a container
3. Cook ground meat until done then add onion and mushroom mixture **4**. Add stewed tomatoes and tomato paste **5**. Add Italian spices, fresh garlic and cook for 3 minutes **6**. Drain all excess liquid and fat **7**. In a large glass casserole dish arrange a thick layer of uncooked spinach. **8**. Followed by a layer of meat mixture, place layer of ricotta cheese and sprinkle shredded cheese.
9. Repeat with layer of meat, ricotta cheese and sprinkle with shredded cheese **10**. Cook in preheated oven at 325 degrees for 1 hour
Let cool for 30-45 minutes before serving
The longer the lasagna is allowed to cool the easier it is to serve

Ginger Chicken Soup
Wonderful on a cold winter day

Ingredients

1 lb skinless cooked chicken cubed or shredded (your choice)
1 inch piece of fresh ginger
1-2 garlic cloves minced.
1/2 teaspoon fish sauce
1/2 cup chopped leeks
6 cups low sodium chicken broth
2 chopped basil leaves
2-3 cups zucchini squash or cabbage
2 teaspoons olive oil.
low sodium bouillon paste

Directions

1. In a small saucepan place olive oil and sauté the leeks and garlic cloves **2**. Meanwhile place the low sodium chicken broth in a medium size pot on medium heat **3**. When broth starts to boil add cooked chicken, fish sauce along with sautéed leeks and garlic cloves **4**. Lower the heat for about 10 minutes and let the flavors mix **5**. Raise heat and let soup come to a boil **6**. Remove from heat and add chopped basil and chopped zucchini. Cover and let sit for 3-5 minutes before serving. Use vegetable or chicken low sodium bouillon paste to add flavor instead of salt.
You may use the broth from the cooked chicken
Hints: if you do not like ginger leave the piece intact and remove before serving.
If you add the zucchini or cabbage too early it overcooks

Baked Lemon Sole

Enjoy

Ingredients

2 garlic cloves
4 lemon sole fillets, about 6oz each
1 shallot, finely chopped
2 fresh lemon thyme sprigs, plus extra to garnish
2 fresh lemon balm sprigs, plus extra to garnish
Salt and pepper to taste
Grated rind and juice of 1 lemon
2 Tablespoons extra virgin olive oil

Directions

1. Using a sharp knife, thinly slice the garlic and set aside
2. Arrange the sole fillets in a single layer in the bottom of an ovenproof dish and sprinkle the shallot **3**. Place the reserve garlic slices and fresh herb sprigs on top of the fillets and season with salt and pepper **4**. Mix the lemon juice and olive oil together in a small measuring cup and pour it over the fish **5**. Bake in oven at 350 for 15 minutes or until the fish easily flakes when tested with a fork
6. Sprinkle with lemon rind, garnish with extra fresh herbs

Diet of Hope Summer Salad

This salad is so versatile it can be eaten on its own or used as a base for other dishes.

Ingredients

1 small tomato, diced
½ small yellow bell pepper, diced
½ small cucumber, diced
¼ cup red onion, diced
1 Tablespoon red wine vinegar
1 teaspoon extra virgin olive oil
Salt and pepper to taste

Directions

1. Dice all ingredients **2**. Combine wine vinegar, olive oil, and salt and pepper in a bowl, mix well **3**. Add vegetables and toss.
Allow to sit in refrigerator for a couple of hours before serving.
This recipe can be doubled for larger serving size

Salmon and Chive Omelet

Health Discover it in your life

Ingredients

2 eggs
1 teaspoon chopped fresh chives or spring onions (scallions)
1teaspoon of butter
1 -1/2 oz of cooked salmon roughly chopped
¼ cup of parsley for garnish

Directions

1. Break the eggs into a bowl and beat with a fork **2.** Stir in the chopped chives or spring onions, season with salt and pepper and set aside **3.** In pan set on low heat, melt the butter **4.** Pour in the eggs and cook for 3-4 minutes **5.** Draw the egg to the center of the pan from time to time **6.** Before removing the egg, top with the salmon and fold the omelet in half and garnish with parsley.

Crunchy Shrimp Chicharron (Pork Rind)

The Pork rind can be used with any meat to give it some crunch

Ingredients

1 lb Shrimp cleaned and deveined
2 eggs whites beaten
3-4 Tablespoons extra virgin olive oil
1 16 oz bag of spicy Chicharrones (pork rinds, found in potato chip aisle)

Directions

1. Place Chicharrones in a plastic bag and pound with mallet until they are finely ground **2**. Take cleaned deveined shrimp and completely coat with egg white mixture **3**. Then transfer them one at time into bag with the ground Chicharron and coat shrimp completely **4**. In a large skillet warm 1-2 Tablespoons of the olive oil, place shrimp in skillet and cook for 3-4 minutes in medium to low heat, or until shrimp Is thoroughly cooked.

The ground chicharron can be used to coat chicken and make chicken fingers. Not everyone likes the spicy ones so you can use regular chicharron.

Hearty Chicken in Red Wine Sauce
Believe in the power of health

Ingredients

2-4 chicken breast
½ cup red wine
¼ cup butter
1 Tablespoon crushed garlic
1 teaspoon black pepper
1 Tablespoon olive oil
2 cups diced bell peppers (use 2 different colors)
1 Tablespoons ground paprika
1 teaspoon salt
1 cup leeks, finely chopped
½ cup low sodium chicken broth

Directions

1. Combine garlic, salt, pepper and paprika and coat chicken **2**. In a skillet put ½ of the olive oil and sauté the leeks and the bell peppers until leeks are translucent **3**. Remove the leeks and bell peppers from the skillet and set aside **4**. Place the rest of the olive oil in the skillet and brown the chicken **5**. Add the low sodium bouillon and cover the skillet for about 8 minutes on low heat **6**. When chicken is completely done, add the leeks peppers and butter and slowly introduce the red wine **7**. Continue to cook for another 2-3 minutes so the flavors blend. (The longer you cook the more the alcohol evaporates)

Hot Beef in Coconut Curry

Health is the recipe for life

Ingredients

¾ cups coconut milk
2 Tablespoons Thai red curry paste
2 garlic cloves crushed
1 lb braising Steak 3-4oz each
2 kaffir lime leaves, shredded
3 Tablespoons Thai fish sauce
½ teaspoon ground turmeric
2 Tablespoon chopped fresh basil leaves
2 Tablespoon chopped fresh cilantro leaves
Salt and pepper to taste
2 teaspoons lemon juice
1 large fresh red chile, deseeded and sliced

Directions

1. Place coconut milk in a large sauce pan and bring to a boil 2. Lower the heat and simmer gently over low heat for about 8-10 minutes until the milk has thickened 3. Stir in the red curry paste and garlic and simmer for another 3-4 minutes 4. Cut beef into ¾ inch chunks, add to the pan and bring to a boil, stirring frequently 5. Lower the heat and add the lime leaves, lime juice, fish sauce, chile, turmeric and ½ teaspoon of salt 6. Cover the pan and simmer gently for another 20-25 minutes or until the sauce dries or gets absorbed 7. Stir in basil and cilantro and add pepper and salt to taste
Serve Hot

BODY MASS INDEX CHART

BMI	19	20	21	22	23	24	25	26
Height				Weight (lbs.)				
4'10"	91	96	100	105	110	115	119	124
4'11"	94	99	104	109	114	119	124	128
5'0"	97	102	107	112	118	123	128	133
5'1"	100	106	111	116	122	127	132	137
5'2"	104	109	115	120	126	131	136	142
5'3"	107	113	118	124	130	135	141	146
5'4"	110	116	122	128	134	140	145	151
5'5"	114	120	126	132	138	144	150	156
5'6"	118	124	130	136	142	148	155	161
5'7"	121	127	134	140	146	153	159	166
5'8"	125	131	138	144	151	158	164	171
5'9"	128	135	142	149	155	162	169	176
5'10"	132	139	146	153	160	167	174	181
5'11"	136	143	150	157	165	172	179	186
6'0"	140	147	154	162	169	177	184	191
6'1"	144	151	159	166	174	182	189	197
6'2"	148	155	163	171	179	186	194	202
6'3"	152	160	168	176	184	192	200	208
6'4"	156	164	172	180	189	197	205	213

BODY MASS INDEX CHART (Continued)

BMI	27	28	29	30	35	40
Height			Weight (lbs.)			
4'10"	129	134	138	143	167	191
4'11"	133	138	143	148	173	198
5'0"	138	143	148	153	179	204
5'1"	143	148	153	158	185	211
5'2"	147	153	158	164	191	218
5'3"	152	158	163	169	197	225
5'4"	157	163	169	174	204	232
5'5"	162	168	174	180	210	240
5'6"	167	173	179	186	216	247
5'7"	172	178	185	191	223	255
5'8"	177	184	190	197	230	262
5'9"	182	189	196	203	236	270
5'10"	188	195	202	207	243	278
5'11"	193	200	208	215	250	286
6'0"	199	206	213	221	258	294
6'1"	204	212	219	227	265	302
6'2"	210	218	225	233	272	311
6'3"	216	224	232	240	279	319
6'4"	221	230	238	246	287	328

RECOMMENDED READING LIST

Good Calories-Bad Calories, Gary Taube. Anchor Books, 2008.
Gary Taubes is a science journalist. He gives us great insight in the controversial science of diet and health, weight control and disease.

Why We Get Fat and What to do About It, Gary Taubes. Anchor Books, 2011. This book is a condensed version of *Good Calories-Bad Calories*.

Fat Chance, Robert H. Lustig, MD. Hudson Street Press, 2012.
Dr. Lustig's You-Tube video "Sugar: The Bitter Truth" has been watched by millions. Dr. Lustig is a pediatric endocrinologist. He has been studying the effect of sugar on the central nervous system, metabolism and disease.

Wheat Belly, William Davis, MD. Rodale Book, 2011.
Dr. Davis practices preventive cardiology. In his book he shares revealing research on the disease-creating effects of modern day wheat.

Eat, Drink and Be Healthy, Walter C. Willett, MD. Fireside, 2002.
Dr. Willett is chairman of the Department of Nutrition at the Harvard School of Public Health. He explains why the USDA food guidelines are not only wrong, but dangerous.

Enter the Zone, Barry Sears, Ph.D. Regan Books, 1995.
Barry Sears is a pioneer in biotechnology. A visionary describing the beneficial effect of eicosanoids the omega fats. He recommends calorie restriction and avoiding simple carbohydrates to get into "the zone."

The Modern Nutritional Diseases, Alice and Fred Ottoboni, Ph.Ds.
Vincente Books, 2002.
Alice and Fred Ottoboni are public health scientists. They have convincing arguments that the modern American heart healthy diet is the cause of modern nutritional diseases.

Fats that Heal and Fats that Kill, Udo Erasmus, Ph.D. Alive Books, 1993.
Dr. Erasmus reveals valuable information about fats and their effects.

The New Atkins for a New You, Eric Westman MD, Stephen D. Phinney MD, Jeff S. Volek Ph.D. Touchstone, 2010.
Eric Westman is the director of the Duke Lifestyle Medicine Clinic. Stephen Phinney is professor of medicine emeritus at the University of California Davis School of Medicine. Jeff Volek is an associate professor in the Department of Kinesiology at the University of Connecticut. This is a great review of the updated science of the Atkins diet.

The End of Overeating, David A. Kessler, MD. Rodale, 2009.
Dr. Kessler is former FDA commissioner. He shares insights into the practices of the food industry.

The Diabetic Diet, Richard K. Bernstein, MD. Little, Brown and Company, 2005.
Dr. Bernstein is a type-1 diabetic who is healthy at age eighty, and is a strong proponent of the low carbohydrate diet.

Dietmar Gann, MD

Dr. Gann was born and raised in Germany. He finished Medical School at the University of Tuebingen in 1966, summa cum laude. He studied Cardiology at the University of Miami, later becoming an Associate Professor of Cardiology and the Director of Intensive Care Units at Mount Sinai Medical Center (1974 to 1979). He published 43 scientific articles and practiced Interventional Cardiology in Tucson Arizona from 1979 to 2010. Dr. Gann pioneered multiple new procedures in Tucson: infusing streptokinase (a clot dissolving medication) in occluded arteries of patients with a heart attack, coronary angioplasty, inserting medicated coronary artery stents, aortic valvuloplasty, dual chamber pacemakers and peripheral atherectomies.

During his cardiology career, he became increasingly concerned about the dietary recommendations of our government and medical societies. High carbohydrate diets promote obesity and diabetes. His own research and experience with his patients convinced him that a low carbohydrate diet with ample consumption of none-starchy vegetables and good fats is the answer to many nutritional diseases, including heart disease.

Dr. Gann later co-founded the Diet of Hope Institute with his wife Elizabeth in 2010. The Institute specializes in nutrition, disease management and prevention. During the past 4 years, they have successfully treated over 5,000 patients with diabetes, obesity, hypertension, heart disease and many other nutritional diseases.

Elizabeth Gann, MBA CNC

Elizabeth was named the National Minority Female Entrepreneur of the United States in 2005. She had created a multi-million dollar company, JanCo Janitorial which she started with one part time employee (herself). She was recognized as the Tucson Hispanic Chamber of Commerce Business Woman of the Year, she received the YWCA Leadership Award, the Ana Maria Arias Award and numerous other awards.

She became interested in nutrition when nearly all the adults of her extended family became diabetics. Her mother died from a diabetic complication where both her legs were amputated. For this reason, Elizabeth decided to study nutrition and became a Certified Nutrition Consultant. Together with her husband Dietmar, she founded the highly successful Dr. Gann's Diet of Hope in 2010.

Elizabeth and her husband enjoy hiking, mountain climbing, all water sports and tennis. Together, they successfully climbed numerous mountains including Mount Elbrus in Russia, Mount Kilimanjaro in Africa and Mount Ararat, in Turkey. Also, Dietmar participated in a trek to the North Pole.